Problems from a S

the Royal College of Psych

Foreword by

Thomas Bewley

dent of the College

Tavistock Publications
London and New York

First published in 1986
by Tavistock Publications Ltd
11 New Fetter Lane, London EC4P 4EE

Published in the USA by
Tavistock Publications
in association with Methuen, Inc.
29 West 35th Street, New York NY 10001

Set by Hope Services, Abingdon
Printed in Great Britain
by Richard Clay (The Chaucer Press) Ltd,
Bungay, Suffolk

British Library Cataloguing in Publication Data

Alcohol: our favourite drug: new report
on alcohol and alcohol-related problems
from a special committee of the Royal
College of Psychiatrists.
1. Alcoholism—Great Britain
I. Royal College of Psychiatrists
362.2'92'0941   HVS446
ISBN 0–422–61110–7
ISBN 0–422–61120–4 Pbk

Library of Congress Cataloging in Publication Data

Royal College of Psychiatrists
Alcohol, Our Favourite Drug.
Prepared by the special committee
on alcohol related problems.
Bibliography: P.
Includes indexes
1. Alcoholism—Great Britain—Congresses.
2. Alcoholics—Great Britain—Psychology—Congresses.
3. Alcohol—physiological effect—Congresses.
I. Royal College of Psychiatrists. Special Committee on
Alcohol-related problems.
II. Title. (DNLM: 1. Alcoholism. WM 2745 R888A)
IIV5444.R68   1986   616.86'1   86–14577
ISBN 0–422–61110–7
ISBN 0–422–61120–4 (PBK)

Contents

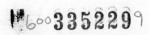

Membership of the special committee on alcohol-related problems

DR J. CHICK

Consultant, Alcohol Problems Clinic, Royal Edinburgh Hospital.
Senior Lecturer, Department of Psychiatry, University of Edinburgh.

PROFESSOR A. W. CLARE

Professor of Psychological Medicine, St Bartholomew's Hospital Medical
College, London.

DR B. D. HORE

Consultant Psychiatrist, Alcoholism Treatment Unit and Detoxification
Centre, Withington Hospital, Manchester (Honorary Lecturer in Psychiatry,
University of Manchester).

PROFESSOR R. E. KENDELL

Professor of Psychiatry, University of Edinburgh.

DR M. Y. MORGAN

Physician, Senior Research Fellow and Honorary Senior Lecturer, The Royal
Free Hospital, London.

DR M. PLANT

Sociologist, Senior Research Fellow, Alcohol Research Group, Department of
Psychiatry, University of Edinburgh.

DR B. RITSON (CHAIRMAN)

Consultant, Alcohol Problems Clinic, Royal Edinburgh Hospital.
Senior Lecturer, Department of Psychiatry, University of Edinburgh.

DR R. J. WAWMAN (OBSERVER)

Principal Medical Officer, with special responsibility in alcohol misuse. Department of Health and Social Security, London.

Acknowledgements

Many people have helped the Committee in preparing this Report. We would particularly like to mention the help received from the Committee of the College chaired by Professor Edwards which prepared the first report (*Alcohol and Alcoholism*). The dependency/addiction group of the Royal College of Psychiatrists also provided helpful advice as did Mr Ian Robertson, Ms Linda Hunt, Professor Norman Kreitman and Dr Moira Plant. Dr Jane Morris gave invaluable assistance in reviewing the text.

We are very grateful to Mrs Patricia Rose and to Mrs Valerie Dunn for the patience and care with which they prepared successive drafts of this Report.

Foreword

Alcohol is the major public health issue of our time, overshadowing even that of tobacco and dwarfing the problems of illicit drug abuse. The Royal College of Psychiatrists published a report, *Alcohol and Alcoholism*, in 1979. The problems associated with the use of alcohol were reviewed and a comprehensive account of the epidemiology, social background, clinical features and management of alcohol dependence was given. That report laid emphasis on the fact that the level of consumption by the whole of the population and the damage to health caused by alcohol were closely associated.

In the fifteen years before the writing of that report the annual per capita consumption of alcohol in the United Kingdom had increased from 5.2 litres to 9.7 litres. This was a cause for grave concern. The College recommended that the per capita consumption by the community at large should not be allowed to rise further and also suggested an upper limit of daily drinking beyond which an individual might expect to be damaged. There was, of course, an implicit assumption that the amount consumed by the majority would have to be substantially below such an 'upper limit' if progress was to be made in the foreseeable future. During the 1970s most indicators of alcohol-related harm had risen steeply in line with the rapid increase in per capita consumption. Since around 1980 most of these trends have reached a plateau, as has consumption, probably in relation to the economic recession.

It is fascinating to study the varying rates of consumption of alcohol in Britain and to relate these to physical, mental and emotional harm. For many years before the First World War the consumption per capita was high. A range of measures to control this (introduced by Lloyd George) led to a pronounced fall in rates of consumption. These remained low until the end of the Second World War. Since then there has been a gradual decrease in the real price of alcohol with a steady increase in the rates of consumption. At the same time there have been large increases in the rates of cirrhosis of the liver, admissions to psychiatric units and mental hospitals for alcoholism, drunkenness offences, drunk driving offences and many other alcohol related harms (such as wife and child battering, violence and accidents).

There is, at present, a very high level of public concern about illicit drug abuse. During 1983, 77 deaths in Britain were attributed to the inhalation of glue and solvents and 82 were attributed to opiates and other illicit drugs. These figures are, of course, disturbing and this College will be producing a report on drug abuse in the near future. Alcohol misuse is, however, annually associated with over 4,000 deaths, 50,000 convictions for drunk driving and 5,000 first admissions to psychiatric hospitals for alcohol dependence and alcoholic psychosis. It is our favourite socially acceptable drug and as such it has many benefits but the costs must be acknowledged and placed in a proper perspective.

In 1982, the Department of Health and Social Security (DHSS) produced a discussion document 'Prevention and Health, Drinking Sensibly'. This reflected some but not all of the recommendations of an earlier unpublished report in 1979 from the Government Central Policy Review Staff ('Think Tank'). These two reports covered similar ground but the differences between them were revealing. The DHSS discussion document did not follow the 'Think Tank' proposal that the trend towards making alcohol relatively cheaper should be arrested. Nor did the DHSS document support the view that there might be a case for the systematic use of tax rates as a means of regulating consumption, though there is ample evidence in the College's own report and other documents that fiscal measures are one of the most effective means of regulating the overall level of per capita consumption and reducing alcohol-related harm.

A number of approaches to containing damage associated with the abuse of alcohol are possible. These include early detection of problem drinkers, which can be encouraged by training courses for general practitioners and social workers and policies in industry for assisting alcohol-impaired employees. Such initiatives are welcome and require development. They will benefit some individuals but they will have little effect on society as a whole. Efforts can also be made to educate the public to 'drink moderately and sensibly'. Although excessive drinkers will reduce their personal risk if they curtail their consumption there numbers are so small that they will have little impact on the public health problem because most casualties are generated by the numerically much larger 'lower risk' consumers in the community. Other campaigns have been directed towards school-children. Their chief difficulties are that the knowledge and attitudes of school-leavers have not been shown to predict their drinking habits a few years later. Knowledge may be enhanced by education while attitudes are untouched and may even be adversely affected. The impact of these programmes is hampered by massive counter-education provided by the media and advertising, all of which constantly encourages drinking. The public health approach is probably the soundest. This seeks to achieve a reduction in national consumption of alcohol. The usual objection to such a policy is that heavy drinkers will continue to drink excessively whatever constraints are imposed. Against this evidence can be cited at length showing that indicators such as liver cirrhosis and even suicide rates vary directly with *average* consumption. Longitudinal studies have shown that when alcohol becomes more expensive and consumption falls, the heavy drinkers reduce their consumption by the same degree as do the light drinkers.

Three groups of strategies could be applied to lower per capita consumption. The most powerful one is the use of fiscal measures, which might be considered to be 'unfair' to poorer people, though this is true of all sales taxes. The second group of measures concern the availability of alcohol. There are issues here not only of supermarket sales but also of the permeation of all aspects of contemporary life by alcohol. The third area concerns advertising and sponsorship. The empirical data is uncertain but some countries have already introduced total bans on alcohol advertising as an experiment. The impact of these developments should be monitored with interest. Such programmes inevitably encounter obstacles. A central difficulty is co-ordination within government where, for instance, one department, the Treasury, is concerned to maximize revenue while another, the Department of Health, is concerned to minimize health problems. Fifteen different government departments have some concern about different aspects of alcohol policy but their plans are insufficiently co-ordinated. There are also understandable conflicts with trade interests and economic considerations which arise from the large number of individuals employed in the drink trade.

The College has reviewed the advice on sensible personal levels of consumption that it gave in its first report. Continuing research has confirmed a greater risk for women who drink heavily, and different guidelines are now needed for each sex. An upper limit above which an individual might expect to be damaged is not a guide to what should be encouraged. Many people do not know what grammes or centilitres of absolute alcohol are equivalent to in terms of individual drinks. For this reason advice is now given in terms of a 'unit' (a single measure of spirits or a half-pint of beer or a glass of wine). It is hoped that by so doing it will be easier for people to review their own pattern of drinking, and also that of their family and friends.

The Royal College of Psychiatrists have been concerned for some time with the many problems associated with dependence on alcohol and other drugs and has recently formed a special section of the College to review and advise how these can best be tackled. There is a serious concern that the services for problem drinkers lack adequate resources and little in the way of real guidelines for the development of services have been produced, despite the reports of the Advisory Committee on Alcoholism which has regrettably been disbanded. Perhaps the single most important point made in this College's first report was the potential harm associated with our increasing use of this drug and the need for greater knowledge of all its effects both good and bad. That report was warmly welcomed and it has now become necessary to provide a further report. This new report builds on the foundations of the first and updates and improves it in the light of further research and knowledge and other reports which have appeared recently. Professor Griffith Edwards and his colleagues should be congratulated for the success of the first report and Dr Bruce Ritson and his co-workers deserve our thanks for re-writing and updating it in its preseent form.

THOMAS BEWLEY
President

1

The need for a further Report

INTRODUCTION

This Report is intended for everyone who has concern with one of the major health and social problems which confronts this and many other nations. As our Report will show, it is a fundamental misunderstanding of the nature of alcohol problems to suppose that they can simply be handed over to doctors and social workers. The people who must share in this concern are the mass of ordinary citizens, as well as a wide range of professionals, and those whose work calls on them to implement local and national policy. The Report is deliberately written in non-technical language, to make it intelligible to the widest possible general readership, as well as to people in the professions that have a part to play. To find a style of expression that will suit the lay person as well as the specialist is notoriously difficult, but if a report is concerned with basic issues rather than with technical details, which are strictly the professional's remit, we believe a common language is possible. For example, the Report will not seek to deal with technical details of treatment such as the choice of drug to combat withdrawal symptoms, or the staffing ratio of an in-patient unit, but on the other hand, it will be concerned to test basic assumptions regarding who is likely to respond to help, or what treatment may achieve.

Part of the intention of this Report is therefore to ask questions, to test assumptions, and to tackle confusions. It aims to inform, and to provide the essential facts on which discussion can be based. Its intention is also to make proposals for a better response to meet these problems – and, as has already been stressed, we believe that what has to be done is the business of that very wide readership which we hope to engage in the necessary debate.

Of course we do not believe that there are suddenly, today, some new and fundamental insights or miraculous technologies which, if properly applied, would at a stroke eliminate a problem that has baffled society for centuries. The Report is intended for those who seek no easy comfort nor spurious slogans but who believe that something better has to be done, and that better actions often require not only compassion and determination but clarity in ideas.

The Royal College of Psychiatrists' first report on *Alcohol and Alcoholism* affirmed the College's concern about the nature and extent of alcohol-related problems in this country. In this book we have revised and updated that Report and taken stock of the responses or lack of responses which have been evident since its publication in 1979. *We have also given this report a title which underlines the fact that alcohol is a drug.* At a time when there is so much public concern about 'drug abuse' we believe it is important to keep in mind that alcohol is our most widely used, and yet most damaging, drug.

Alcohol is a substance which most of the time is used wisely and well by the majority of people who drink and who derive pleasure and benefit from its use. Alcohol is also a drug, which, if misused, can miserably wreck or destroy life, and which exacts these costs on a devastating scale.

Given the equal truth of these two statements it is not surprising that a balanced perspective on alcohol has so far eluded society's grasp. The obvious reaction is to fly to extremes. Some people may be resentful, or resistant, when confronted with forceful evidence about the human costs of a substance which gives them pleasure and the use of which is deeply embedded in convivial custom. The tendency will be to dismiss the casualties as few in number, and to stigmatize them as undeserving; they are said to be the over-indulgent fringe who can give any pleasure a bad name, besides which their wounds are self-inflicted. In this way people who have been harmed by drink are disregarded. Alternatively, the problem can be tidied away with an appearance of greater generosity by regarding those who develop alcohol-related problems as sick rather than bad: their drinking is symptomatic of underlying illness, and they must be handed over to the medical profession for treatment. With this sad minority thus kindly dealt with, the rest of us may, with good conscience, go on our drinking way unworried. Whether the excessive drinker is labelled as bad or ill, society all too readily neutralizes its own anxieties.

The contrary reaction, though certainly not the one that wins the majority vote, is to exaggerate the dangers of alcohol and see its use as an unmitigated evil. Drinking itself becomes the devil to be cast out of individuals and society alike. Neither of these extreme reactions serves society well. Their harm lies not only in misleading individuals about their own or their neighbour's drinking, but also in misinforming large-scale national policies. The extreme results can then be either the excesses of Gin Lane, or the excesses of Prohibition.

The fundamental purpose of this Report is to develop a perspective on alcohol and alcohol problems which avoids either extreme; a perspective which is based on the most recent evidence but which admits gaps in information where these exist; and which may then accurately serve the needs of the individual, the professional, and the designer of public policies, in a society where alcohol is likely to remain a favoured recreational drug.

TIME TO RESPOND TO A LARGE AND THREATENING PROBLEM

A major reason for the existence of this second Report is the mass of data which continues to demonstrate the seriousness of the drinking problems that society is facing. The Report deals not with a minor and peripheral social ill, worthy of attention only when there is a little reforming energy to spare, but with an endemic disorder of frightening magnitude.

Indeed, the question as to 'the sum of damage' demands an outline answer immediately, although a full account must be delayed until later. The plain fact is that problems of alcohol misuse constitute an appalling insult to the nation's health, a cause of untold personal and family misery and a cost to the country measured in thousands of millions of pounds each year. Such a statement might be thought to call into question the objectivity of this Report, but there is ample factual evidence to support it and to show that it is in no way an exaggeration. We shall give a brief synopsis in the next few paragraphs of some information about damage due to alcohol which will be treated at greater length in Chapter 6.

At a conservative estimate there are at least 300,000 people in this country with drinking problems of such severity as to merit the conventional label of 'alcohol dependence', and this may well be an underestimate. In 1978, a survey of drinking in England and Wales found that 5 per cent of men and 2 per cent of women reported alcohol-related problems. Each of these people is probably affecting the health, happiness, or safety of several family members, friends, and workmates. People with serious drinking problems have an expectation of dying which is between two and three times greater than that of members of the general population of the same age and sex. Recent research in general hospitals showed that approximately 25 per cent of acute male admissions to medical wards were directly or indirectly due to alcohol misuse, and an even higher proportion of acute surgical emergencies proved to be abnormal drinkers. Annual admissions to psychiatric hospitals for treatment of alcohol dependence have increased more than twenty-five-fold in the last twenty-five years and now exceed 17,500 per year in England and Wales: the cost of psychiatric hospital care alone must now be upwards of £17 million per annum. It is estimated that non-psychiatric medical care costs a further £50 million at least.

That figure is small by comparison with the non-medical cost of excessive drinking: the Blennerhasset Committee on drunk driving estimated in 1976 that the annual costs of road traffic accidents due to drinking must be about £100 million each year, and drunk driving has increased steeply since that time. A current estimate of the cost in terms of money alone is of the order of £178 million. In Britain, approximately 100,000 drunkenness arrests are now taken annually through the courts. Drink is implicated in the offences of about 60 per cent of the petty recidivists who contribute so largely to the prison population; notwithstanding concern about drug-related crime, without the problems of excessive drinking the courts would suddenly be underemployed and the prisons remarkably uncrowded. The costs of alcohol misuse to industry, and the costs in terms of welfare and sickness benefits are certainly enormous. Economists have estimated that in 1983 the social costs related to alcohol misuse in the United Kingdom were £1,614 millions.

As for the impact on the family, the husband's excessive drinking seems to be implicated in not less than 50 per cent of cases of wife-battering. The impact of drinking on the psychological development of the children of problem drinkers is painfully evident to teachers, social workers, paediatricians and social workers.

The evidence is not only that a problem of great size exists, but one which in nearly every aspect has increased markedly over the past twenty years. There has been until very recently continuous escalation in such available indices of alcohol misuse as deaths from cirrhosis, hospital admissions for alcoholism, drunkenness arrests, and drunk driving arrests. Underlying these separate changes there is the basic fact that the nation is drinking much more: from 1950 to 1980 the alcohol consumption per head of the adult population approximately doubled. Consumption peaked in 1979, there was a slight fall between 1980 and 1982, probably associated with economic recession and price increases, but the level rose in 1983 and again in 1984. There was a welcome decline in drunkenness offences between 1980 and 1983 but the level remains far higher than it was earlier this century. Although each indicator, taken individually, may be a somewhat uncertain pointer (there can be distortions introduced by such factors as change in diagnostic awareness or in police practice), taken all together the evidence that the problem has grown steadily greater over recent decades is incontrovertible (see Chapter 2).

In addition to the general rise in the country's experience of alcohol-related problems, there is much to suggest that within the total population certain groups are now more heavily affected than before. For instance, some teachers report that alcohol misuse has become a major school-age problem, and they have to deal with children who have been drinking in the lunch hour. Official figures show that convictions for drunkenness among teenagers have more than doubled since 1964. In 1984 the age at which the rate of individual offending was highest was eighteen for both males and females. Cirrhosis of the liver is becoming more common in younger age groups. There is also much evidence that drinking problems among women are on the increase.

The increase in alcohol-related problems should not necessarily be taken as proof positive that alcohol dependence rates are immediately going to surge further out of control. It is possible that over the next few years, and with a standstill or actual fall in real wages and less money to spend on drink, there could be some temporary diminution in drinking problems. There was evidence of some plateauing of the level of problems in the early 1980s, although they remained at an unacceptably high level, so that efforts to win the nation's concern by incautious scare-mongering may lose rather than capture public attention.

The position adopted here is that the threat posed by all these ominous pointers should neither be discounted nor exaggerated, but the information available should remind us that there is no guarantee of immunity from further and explosive increases in these problems. France has for many years had a death rate from cirrhosis about ten times that in Britain; over the next fifty years, and with all the benefits of closer integraton with continental Europe, we cannot rule out the possibility that drinking and drinking problems will reach uniform and high levels throughout Europe. Who for instance is going to drink the 'wine lake' of surplus EEC production? Many old socio-cultural, legal, and economic barriers may disappear by the end of the century as may the barriers that have for centuries determined the individuality of different national drinking patterns. If unchecked by any insistence on

health considerations, economic interests might well promote a new
level of pan-European problem drinking, a level located nearer that of
the countries such as France, Italy and Germany with the highest
incidence of alcohol-related problems.

In summary, the facts substantiate the conclusion that the problem
which we already have remains sufficiently serious to constitute an
immediate cause for concern. If the casualty rates were to dip to the
lowest level recorded in this century, they would still be worrying. If,
on the other hand, emancipated adolescents were to drink more like
adults, more liberated women were to drink more like men, and
Britons, having become good Europeans, were to drink more like the
French, then there are threats which are potentially appalling.

CATCHING A TIDE OF AWARENESS

Over the last two decades there has been an improvement in this
country's awareness of its drinking problems. The nature of some of
these developments is charted in Chapter 3. But the very fact of this
new activity sets problems. There is the danger of energies being
misspent, and of policies being firmly adopted and implemented
without sufficient thought being given to the options. One of the
reasons for this second Report is that despite the debates and
discussion documents of the past decade the country lacks a clear and
coherent response to drinking problems. The issues have become
clearer, some methods have been tested, but cause for serious concern
persists. If the opportunity is not now seized, options will be closed and
a time for beneficial action will have been lost.

Time to identify the confusions

When few people in the country were particularly concerned about
alcohol problems, a deceptive clarity of views could be assumed to exist
– each side could hold its extreme and straightforward position
unchallenged. But varieties of confusion have come about, or have
come into sharper focus, as a by-product of the greater interest now
taken in drinking problems. It is timely to attempt to identify these
confusions (even if they cannot all be resolved), rather than only half-
recognizing them when they can persist as pitfalls in planning and
social action (see pp. 36–7).

Time to capitalize on new knowledge

There would not be much point in writing a report if nothing more
could be done than itemize the problems and list the confusions. On

the contrary, and very fortunately, it should be eminently possible to tackle some of these difficulties in ways not possible before, armed with insights which have come from new knowledge on alcohol and alcohol-related problems gained in recent years. This knowledge bears on such questions as the nature of alcohol dependence, why people drink or drink excessively, and the social, economic and cultural influences on rates of alcohol misuse. But also to be noted is a serious and widening gap which some have calculated as twenty years between what is known and the use that is being made of the information now readily to hand. Policies on prevention and treatment have been substantially revised but lack the commitment and support to develop new approaches except in a piecemeal way. The time has come to examine the ways in which new knowledge can lead to a restructuring of the nation's response.

THE MEANING OF TERMS

For our present purposes, we do not need a greatly detailed theoretical analysis of these problems of definition. A set of ideas and criteria is essential, however, to serve the practical needs of communication, so that when two people talk about matters dealt with in this Report they will be talking about roughly the same things. In the ordinary world a lot of communication constantly centres on abnormal drinking: a wife debating with her husband whether he is or is not an 'alcoholic'; the doctor trying to establish a diagnosis and communicate with his or her patient; the expression by a psychiatrist or social worker of a professional opinion and the court's attempt to understand exactly what is implied by the technically-worked statement; and the facts and arguments being presented to the public on alcohol and health. Because people of many different backgrounds have to find words for communicating with each other, the critical need is for a set of clear definitions which are understood by different professions, and by the world in general.

With this purpose in mind, a brief exposition of the ideas and definitions used in this Report will be given below. These ideas will be taken further in each of the following chapters; here, only an outline will be given. Our presentation will borrow freely from a World Health Organisation publication (*Alcohol-Related Disabilities*, 1977) which tried to meet the challenge of designing a framework of ideas not only to serve the needs of communication between different people in the same country, but also to aid communication between individuals in different countries.

alcoholism' is in common use, but at the same time there
ertainty about its meaning. Where is the dividing line
drinking and this 'illness'? Is it a matter of quantity
..ge sustained, or addiction, or of what else besides? This
..inusion is not limited to the lay person, for final clarification has
eluded the many experts and expert committees that have grappled
with the terms used to describe drinking problems.

Alcohol dependence

Alcohol is, in familiar terms, a drug of 'addiction'. The word
'addiction', having fallen out of favour in discussions of drinking in
recent years because of its association with narcotic use, has been
replaced by the term 'dependence'. The hallmark of dependence is an
inability to refrain from taking alcohol without experiencing psychological
and/or physical discomfort. The nature of dependence on alcohol will
be considered carefully in Chapter 5, and the very serious personal and
social implications will be discussed there and in Chapter 6. It is vital
that there should be general and full understanding about the severe
and harmful dependence that can be associated with our society's most
favoured recreational drug.

Alcohol-related disabilities

Although the reality of the phenomenon of alcohol dependence needs
to be brought very much to public attention, it must also be underlined
that the use of alcohol can result in a host of other physical, social, and
mental disabilities (Chapter 6). Anyone who is severely dependent is
likely to incur serious alcohol-related disabilities and, because of
diminished ability to modify their drinking in the face of such
punishing experience, they will go on incurring more and more harm.
To this extent dependence and disability march hand-in-hand – it is
almost impossible to imagine someone who is severely dependent who
will not in time incur health or social disabilities as a result of their
drinking.

However, the reverse does not necessarily hold. It is frequently the
case that individuals who are not alcohol dependent none the less use
alcohol in such a way as to damage themselves. It would be entirely
insufficient to view society's alcohol problems such as absenteeism
from work or road traffic accidents exclusively in terms of the number
of people suffering from dependence (and the count of their
disabilities). Such a limited focus has in the past often handicapped
society's appraisal of the problem confronting it: as a result of a too-
narrow concern with dependence, we have forgotten that alcohol to a

greater or lesser extent has adverse impact on the lives of many other people. We need an awareness of the great range of difficulties which may result from drinking, of the less dramatic as well as the dramatic damage. We need to grasp the importance of the many forms of damage to health and to social functioning caused by heavy drinking – whether or not the individual has become dependent on alcohol – and without either disregarding or over-emphasizing dependence where it exists. In strict logic, dependence on alcohol might itself best be seen as one very particular type of disability.

At this point it may be useful to give two excerpts from illustrative case histories:

(a) A man, aged fifty, lost control of his car when drunk and crashed into a lamp-post. He had certainly incurred disabilities; he lost his licence, and broke his leg. The history revealed, however, that he only drank occasionally, but had that evening gone out to dinner with friends and drunk an unaccustomedly large amount. He was not dependent on alcohol, although as a consequence of his drinking he nearly killed himself and might well have killed someone else.

(b) Another man, aged fifty, was on the same night stopped by the police because he was driving slowly and with over-elaborate caution. He was found to have a grossly elevated blood-alcohol level, and was, after prosecution, duly disqualified from driving. He had in fact been disqualified on two previous occasions (and had also been involved in one nasty accident of the hit-and-run variety). If a doctor examined him, this man would be found to have a severely enlarged liver. His wife had left him because of his drinking. He was severely dependent on alcohol and was persistently drinking more than a bottle of whisky each day. He was unable to modify or control his drinking, which increasingly threatened disaster.

In terms of the thinking of this Report, both these men were manifesting behaviour that should have been of the gravest concern to themselves, and to society. To be unconcerned about the first man because he was not alcohol dependent would be to close our eyes to what in sum may be enormously important consequences of drink to society. A story such as the second man gives is, however, also of great importance. No good is served by arguing which man's story is more or less worrying – the implications of both these stories must be of concern.

Alcoholism

The term 'alcoholism' figured prominently in the previous report but has now been largely discarded and used only when it has been employed as a descriptive term in earlier research reports. It is a word that has been used variously by different people and groups and is of imprecise meaning. The fact that much uncertainty attaches to the word is an additional reason for adopting the terms 'dependence' and 'disability'. For most people 'alcoholism' is perhaps synonymous with severe alcohol dependence or 'the disease of alcoholism', and this is probably its usage by Alcoholics Anonymous. For others the term has much more inclusive meaning, embracing every type of instance where someone is incurring serious or persistent disability as a result of his or her drinking, irrespective of dependence. Unfortunately, it has also become an everyday term of abuse. The very unsavoury stereotype which it often conjures up in the mind of the problem drinker may prevent or delay their decision to seek help.

'Alcoholism' as a portmanteau word containing the diverse range of alcohol-related problems that concern us here has certain attractions but it was rejected principally because it is too easy to believe that public concern need focus only on unfortunates who suffer from 'alcoholism' while the rest of us can carry on drinking with impunity. As this Report will show there is no justification for such a comfortable belief.

We believe that some better agreement on how words in this area are to be used would serve not only professional people and administrators, but also the person in the street, the writer of radio or television programmes, and the audience who listen to those programmes. Any terms we adopt today may well be in need of revision in five or ten years' time.

2
A historical perspective

Of all the drugs which human beings have used and abused in the course of their chequered history alcohol is almost certainly the oldest, and also the most widely used, because it is so easily produced. Airborne yeasts readily lead to fermentation in any sugary juice – from grapes, fruit, or berries – if it is exposed to warm air for a few days, and most preliterate peoples soon learnt the intoxicating effects of such juices and how to facilitate the fermentation process. Many also learnt at an early stage how to convert starch containing cereals like maize to alcoholic brews by chewing the cereal and then spitting it into water, which allows salivary amylase to convert the starch to sugars, which yeasts then convert to alcohol.

Alcoholic beverages were well known to most of the early human civilizations. Prescriptions for beer were written on clay tablets by Sumerian physicians more than 2000 years BC and by 1500 BC the papyri of Egyptian doctors included beer or wine in about 15 per cent of their prescriptions. The Hindu Ayurveda, which dates from about 1000 BC, describes the uses of alcoholic beverages and also the consequences of intoxication and habitual intoxication. The oldest surviving code of laws, that of Hammurabi in about 1770 BC, regulated Babylonian drinking houses, and the Semitic cuneiform literature of the pre-Biblical Canaanites contains numerous references to the many religious and household uses of alcohol.

Because of their remarkable effects on behaviour and mood, alcoholic beverages were widely used in religious ceremonies from an early stage, and were often invested with a special religious significance. Wine and beer were both used as offerings to deities of many kinds and as a means of enabling priests and shamans to reach the requisite state of ecstasy or frenzy. Sometimes, of course, they drank too much, and the prophet Isaiah was driven to complain: 'Priest and prophet are addicted to strong drink and bemused with wine; clamouring in their cups, confirmed topers, hiccuping in drunken stupor; every table is covered with vomit.'

But despite Isaiah's strictures wine retained its sacerdotal role in the Hebrews' religion and subsequently for Christianity too. Equating red wine with blood and the symbolic drinking of wine in the Christian Eucharist both arose out of a long tradition which still has many parallels in other cultures and religions. The role of wine was just as prominent in the religion of the ancient Greeks and their Roman successors as it was for the Hebrews. Drinking and drunkenness are recurring themes in Greek mythology and the worship of Dionysus, or Bacchus, the wine god, played a prominent part in the life of the peoples of the Mediterranean for a thousand years. The god's female devotees, the Maenads, worshipped him in drunken orgies and his festival, the Bacchanalia, survives as a contemporary term for a drunken orgy.

It was the religious uses of alcohol which first generated uncontrolled intoxication and drunkenness and by and large it fell to religions to control the dangerous excesses to which alcohol gave rise. Islam in the seventh century AD chose total prohibition. The Qur'ān condemned the use of wine and the disciples of Muhammad ensured that this taboo was respected in all the lands they conquered. A similar process was repeated a thousand years later when a number of ascetic Protestant sects, first in Northern Europe and then in North America, made abstinence a fundamental tenet, derived in their eyes from Biblical ideology just as that of the Muslim was derived from the Qur'ān. Similar sequences of events took place in other parts of the world. The devout adherents of the Buddhist religion, which arose in India in the fifth and sixth centuries BC and spread across southern and eastern Asia, have abstained from alcohol ever since and Hindu Brahmins have done the same. Indeed, on a global scale it is striking how nearly all the successful attempts to control the abuse of alcohol have been based on religious tenet rather than on secular fiat. The history of China, whose main religions never proscribed the use of alcohol, includes several abortive attempts at control or prohibition. Only the pre-Columbian Indians of North America, the Melanesian and Polynesian peoples of the Pacific, and the Aboriginal peoples of Australia remained immune to these conflicts and dilemmas, for only they and a few scattered groups elsewhere did not discover the secret of fermentation (which is probably why the 'firewater' to which the Europeans introduced them had such disastrous effects).

Although it has always been the most widely available, because it can be made from any source of sugar or starch, alcohol is only one of a wide variety of psychoactive substances which have been discovered in the vegetable world. At various times and places the effects of opium (from the immature fruits of the opium poppy), of cannabis (from the Indian hemp plant), of nicotine (from the leaves of the tobacco plant), of caffeine (from the coffee bean or the leaves of the tea bush), of cocaine (from the South American coca plant), of mescalin (from the peyote cactus), and many other substances less well known in contemporary industrial societies have been discovered and then exploited. Some of these drugs have remained in purely local use, like Khat (which contains an amphetamine-like drug, cathinone) in Ethiopia and the Yemen and betel nut in India; others have spread far and wide.

Anyone familiar with the history of humanity's relationship with psychoactive substances cannot fail to be struck by two things. The first is the capacity for finding and then systematically eating, drinking, chewing, or smoking substances with stimulant, euphoriant, or intoxicating properties. No other species behaves in this way, though many have ready access to the plants in question. Nor is this obviously because the human nervous system is fundamentally different from that of other mammals, for under laboratory conditions animals like rats and mice can be made dependent upon the same range of substances (alcohol, nicotine, opiates, barbiturates, etc.) as humans, and will work, persistently and single-mindedly, to obtain further doses.

The second equally striking aspect of this phenomenon is the strong feelings, sometimes laudatory and sometimes condemnatory, which human societies characteristically develop about these various psycho-active substances. All of them are capable of inducing pleasurable subjective states of various kinds. If that were not so no one would take any interest in them. Many, though not all, of them are capable of producing states of dependence (see Chapter 5) in regular users. Many, and perhaps all, have other overtly harmful effects, either medical (i.e. to the health of the user) or social (by inducing irresponsible or antisocial behaviour of varous kinds), or both. All these substances, in other words, have potential attractions at least to the users and most if not all have disadvantages to the users or the society to which they belong. It is not surprising, therefore, that human societies, confronted for the first time with users of one of these substances, have sometimes been uncertain whether to approve or to disapprove. Even tea was anathematized as a 'most deadly poison' by many English physicians when it was first popularized in the early nineteenth century. Nor is it surprising that societies have sometimes changed their opinion in the light of their increasing experience of the drug's effects, as we did in the case of tea. But the strength of feeling involved and the unpredictability of the accompanying judgements, both of individuals and governments, is often very remarkable.

Tobacco was introduced to Europe from the Americas in the second half of the sixteenth century and in England the smoking habit began to spread rapidly towards the end of the century. Smokers themselves were very enthusiastic about the benefits. Robert Burton described it thus: 'Tobacco, divine, rare, super excellent tobacco, which goes far beyond all their panaceas, potable gold, and philosopher's stones, a sovereign remedy to all diseases.' His King, however, took a different view. To James I smoking was: 'A custom loathsome to the eye, harmful to the brain, dangerous to the lungs, and in the black stinking fume thereof, nearest resembling the horrible Stygian smoke of the pit that is bottomless.'

Many other seventeenth-century princes shared his views. In Russia the Tzar Michael Federovitch executed anyone on whom tobacco was found and his successor Alexei Mikhailovitch decreed that anyone caught in possession of tobacco should be tortured until he revealed the name of the supplier. In Turkey the nose of a tobacco user was pierced through with the stem of his pipe and he was ridden through town on a donkey. In the German principality of Luneberg the death penalty for smoking remained in force until 1691.

While European kings and emperors denounced the American drug tobacco and punished its users with the utmost severity their American counterparts denounced alcohol and meted out dire punishments to those who dared to drink it. According to Calderon Narvaez the pre-Hispanic emperor of Mexico addressed his people thus immediately after his election:

'This is the wine known as "octli", which is the root and source of all evil and of all perdition, because octli and drunkenness are the cause of all this discord and strife, and all the rebelliousness and restlessness among the people and Kingdoms; it is like a whirlwind that stirs up and smashes everything; it is like a tempest in hell that brings everything bad with it. Drunkenness is the cause of all the adulteries, rapes, corruption of virgins, and fights with relatives and friends; drunkenness is the cause of all the thefts and robberies and banditry and violence; it is also the cause of cursing and lying and gossip and slander, and of clamouring, quarrels, and shouting.'

Drunkenness in Mexico was therefore treated very severely and savagely punished:

'If a young man appeared in public in a drunken state, or if he was found in possession of wine, or if he was found lying in the street, or singing, or in the company of other drunkards, this young man, if he was a plebeian, was punished by being beaten with clubs until he was dead, or he was garotted in the presence of all the young men, who were gathered together so that this would serve as an example for them.'

Many Western governments now regard heroin and cocaine in much the same light as the Mexican emperor regarded the wine 'octli'. Even cannabis is rigorously proscribed. Its possession is a criminal offence in most industrial countries, and it is subject in international law to the same draconian controls as heroin. In 1953 the United States Commissioner of Narcotics, who was presumably in a position to be well informed on the subject, described cannabis in these terms:

'Marijuana is only and always a scourge which undermines its victims and degrades them mentally, morally, and physically. . . . A small dose taken by one subject may bring about intense intoxification, raving fits, criminal assaults. . . . It is this unpredictable effect which makes marijuana one of the most dangerous drugs known . . . the moral barricades are broken down and often debauchery and sexuality result . . . where mental instability is inherent, the behaviour is generally violent. . . . Constant use produces an incapacity for work and a disorientation of purpose. The drug has a corroding effect on the body and on the mind, weakening the entire physical system and often leading to insanity after prolonged use.'

The legislative counterpart to these extremist views is a forty-year penalty in some United States states merely for possessing cannabis. Yet tens of thousands of young people, many of them intelligent and in other respects law abiding, smile at such views, ignore the penalties and use cannabis just as they do alcohol, as an occasional recreational drug.

Our governments did not always take so stern a view of these drugs, however. Until 1868 both opium and cannabis could be bought perfectly legally in Britain, not only from pharmacists but even from grocers' shops, and the main purpose of the Pharmacy Act of 1868 was to ensure that only pure opium was sold, and only by qualified pharmacists, rather than seriously to restrict access to the drug.

Towards the end of the nineteenth century, however, the British Government was forced to decide what stance it should adopt towards the benefits or dangers of both cannabis and opium because millions of the Queen's Indian subjects used one or other of these drugs regularly and openly. With characteristic Victorian energy and seriousness of purpose formal commissions were set up to advise the government. The seven volume report of the Indian Hemp Commission, published in 1894, concluded that there was little cause for concern:

> 'Viewing the subject generally, it may be added that the moderate use of these drugs is the rule, and that the excessive use is comparatively exceptional. The moderate use practically produces no ill-effects. . . . The excessive use may certainly be accepted as very injurious, though it must be admitted that in many excessive consumers the injury is not clearly marked. The injury done by the excessive use is, however, confined almost exclusively to the consumer himself; the effect on society is rarely appreciable. It has been the most striking feature in this enquiry to find how little the effects of hemp drugs have obtruded themselves on observation. The large number of witnesses of all classes who professed never to have seen these effects, the vague statements made by many who professed to have observed them, the very few witnesses who could recall a case as to give any definite account of it, and the manner in which a large proportion of these cases broke down on the first attempt to examine them, are facts which combine to show most clearly how little injury society has hitherto sustained from hemp drugs.'

The report of the Royal Commission on Opium, also in seven volumes and published only a few months later, was equally reassuring:

> 'Our conclusions, therefore, are that the use of opium among the people of India in British Provinces is, as a rule, a moderate use, and that excess is exceptional, and condemned by public opinion. . . . We have no hesitation in saying that no extended physical or moral degradation is caused by the habit.'

Twentieth-century commentators have suggested that the views of the Royal Commission were coloured by its concern to preserve the very considerable revenues derived by the Government of India from the export of opium to China. Perhaps they were. But they were probably also coloured by the ready availability and widespread use of opiates in Britain itself. For much of the nineteenth century the opium poppy was legally grown and harvested in East Anglia and opium could be bought in chemists' shops as easily as aspirin is now. Laudanum, an alcoholic extract of raw opium, was one of the most widely used of medicines, taken for fevers, for colic, for nervous exhaustion, and even for fun. Fretful babies were calmed with Mother Bailey's Quietening Syrup and unwanted babies were quietened for ever with laudanum by desperate women in working-class slums.

Several things are apparent from this Babel of violent opinions and conflicting policies. First and most obviously, almost every psychoactive drug known to humanity, from alcohol to opium, has been regarded by some government and society as a dire threat to public order and moral standards and by another government and another society as a source of harmless pleasure. It is also clear that a nation and its government may, within the course of a generation or two, change its views completely, so that a drug which at one time was regarded as dangerous and degrading is at another time – sometimes earlier, sometimes later – widely accepted and freely traded and enjoyed. When such changes occur they can often be related to commercial and economic interests. Parliament's attitude to tobacco in the seventeenth century changed abruptly when it became clear that tobacco exports were vital to the survival of the Virginian colonies, and the government which accepted the Report of the Royal Commission on Opium in 1895 was profiting handsomely from a trade in opium which had lost its importance by the time its successor signed the Hague Convention (which proscribed all trading except under close governmental supervision and for strictly medicinal purposes) seventeen years later.

There is another important conclusion to be drawn from the history of cultural attitudes and governmental policies towards psychoactive drugs. Almost every society has at least one drug whose use is tolerated and to a greater or lesser extent institutionalized, sometimes in a religious, sometimes in a purely secular framework. The drugs of other cultures, however, are generally viewed in a quite different light. They are regarded with deep suspicion, and often they are banned and savage penalties imposed on anyone who dares to use them. The Mexican Indians who disapproved so strongly of alcohol had no objections to the potent hallucinogen mescaline which they obtained from the flowering heads of the peyote cactus. Most of the Muslim cultures which have forbidden any use of alcohol for the last thousand years have tolerated the use of cannabis and many had no objections to opium either. And, of course, the Europeans who reacted so violently to the introduction of tobacco in the sixteenth and seventeenth centuries, and of cannabis and heroin in the twentieth century, had few qualms about alcohol.

The reason is quite simple. Alcohol is the chosen intoxicant of European peoples as it has been in many other parts of the world. It has been part of our lives from the very beginnings of our civilization and it is woven inextricably into our culture. Over the years it has acquired innumerable different roles and functions. We drink at Christmas and the New Year, at birthdays and anniversaries, at weddings and funerals. We drink, as others have done before us, to celebrate and symbolize the most fundamental beliefs of our religion. We also drink to celebrate more personal triumphs, and to drown our sorrows too. We drink to give ourselves an appetite, to help us relax, to mark the end of the working day, to prove that we are grown-up, to assert our virility, to help us get to sleep. The list is almost endless. We use the offer of a drink as a symbol of friendship or of gratitude, to seal a bargain, or to mark the end of a quarrel. We toast our monarch, our institutions, and our friends with alcohol. The waiter's or the porter's tip is his 'pourboire' and the gift-wrapped bottle has become a convenient all-purpose present, a suitable means of thanking one's hostess or one's doctor, a birthday present for an uncle or a Christmas gift for a business associate.

Because alcohol is our own chosen, familiar intoxicant, and perhaps also because many people's livelihoods and important economic interests are involved, we do our best to ignore its ill effects, the damage it inflicts on individuals, on families, and at times on the fabric of our society. When someone else's drinking has terrible consequences we tell ourselves that they were fools to drink so much, or that they never could hold their liquor, or that they should have realized they were heading for trouble long ago. Whatever the precise rationalization it is the drinker rather than the drink itself that we blame. Our attitudes to cannabis, cocaine, opium, and heroin are very different. These are alien drugs, imported from distant continents, and we are easily persuaded that they are dangerous. If a student crashes his car after an evening smoking 'pot', if a young man is found dead in a tenement with an empty syringe beside him, if a debutante commits suicide after experimenting with cocaine, we draw quite different conclusions. These tragedies are evidence not so much of the weakness, the folly, or the misfortune of the individuals concerned but of the pernicious dangers and degrading effects of the alien drug.

This striking difference in attitudes to the familiar institutionalized drug and its alien counterparts is not limited to Western societies. In Asia and the Muslim world the situation is, or used to be, almost identical except, of course, that the institutionalized drug was cannabis or opium and the dangerous alien drug the various alcoholic beverages European traders or settlers brought with them. Because alcohol happened to be the favoured intoxicant of Europeans and their colonial descendents in the Americas, and because the political influence of Europe and North America was so strong in the first half of the twentieth century, it was European and American customs, prejudices, and economic interests which determined the policies of the League of Nations and the United Nations rather than the prejudices and economic interests of India, China, and Saudi Arabia. The fact that international traders in cannabis and the opiates have been condemned ever since 1912 as 'traffickers', and subject to weighty penalties, while international trade in alcoholic beverages is not subject to any controls at all, or even monitored, is not the result of any rational appraisal of the pharmacological properties of the drugs concerned, or of any dispassionate comparison of their relative dangers. It is simply the result of the ability of Western Europeans to impose their assumptions, customs, and prejudices on other people.

But although alcohol has been Europe's chosen intoxicant for two or three thousand years its use, and attitudes to its use, have varied greatly from time to time and place to place. The fact that only in southern Europe is the climate mild enough in winter and hot enough in summer for vines to flourish has been a decisive influence from an early stage. For wine became the staple alcoholic drink of Mediterranean and central European countries while their neighbours to the north had to make do with beer, augmented from the sixteenth century onwards, as the technology of distillation improved, by distilled spirits of various kinds. This difference between north and south was accentuated by the Reformation. The Protestants of northern Europe regarded the Church of Rome as corrupt and self-indulgent, and drunkenness was one of many forms of indulgence the Puritans and other reforming sects regarded with disfavour. This moral disapproval was strongly reinforced early in the eighteenth century by alarm at the dramatic ill effects of distilled liquors like the Dutch spirit genever (known as gin by the English), for northern European countries like Holland and England were quicker both to develop the technology of commercial distillation and also to produce the mercantile and industrial towns in which the ill effects of their consumption were most readily apparent. As a result northern European attitudes to alcohol have, for the last three hundred years, been consistently less tolerant of alcohol than those of the Latin peoples further south. Wine has always been regarded as a basic food, like bread, cheese, and olive oil, by the predominantly agricultural societies of southern Europe, and their Catholic religion has usually taken a more charitable view of drunkenness than of other human frailties. In Britain and Scandinavia, on the other hand, several branches of the Protestant church committed themselves to abstinence much as the Muslim faith had a thousand years before, and their preachers often devoted more sermons to the curse of drink than to the other six deadly sins combined. The temperance movement of the nineteenth century was almost exclusively Protestant in origin (and in England largely non-conformist) and all the countries which adopted Prohibition in the 1920s – the United States and most of Canada, Finland, Norway, and Sweden – were mainly or exclusively Protestant. The only Canadian province which did not commit itself to Prohibition was Catholic and French-speaking Quebec, and it was Italian Catholic immigrants who were primarily responsible for the failure of Prohibition in the United States.

Even within our own northern European and predominantly Protestant society attitudes to alcohol and consumption levels have varied greatly from generation to generation. Because excise duty has been levied on alcoholic beverages continuously since 1643 (when Parliament first imposed a tax on beer to help finance its war with Charles I) there are fairly accurate records of English consumption, or at least of legal production and importation, going back to the seventeenth century (though not, unfortunately, to before 1684, so we do not know how effective the disapproval of the Puritans was in curbing actual consumption). It is apparent from these records and numerous contemporary accounts, that consumption, both of individual beverage types and of alcoholic beverages as a whole, has fluctuated greatly in the course of the last three hundred years. In the seventeenth and eighteenth centuries beer consumption per head of population was far higher than it has ever been in the nineteenth or twentieth centuries, partly because in most places it was less likely to be contaminated with sewage than the water supply. The tavern and the church were the two focal points of every community and drunkenness was commonplace. As Dr Johnson once remarked while reminiscing about his boyhood, 'all the decent people in Lichfield got drunk every night, and were not the worse thought of'. Although this indulgent attitude may well have been coloured by his own partiality for drinking and taverns it is important to appreciate that at that time rural drunkenness posed little threat to society. A drunkard in charge of a scythe was much less dangerous, at least to others, than a drunkard in charge of a steam pump or a motorcar, and the hazards to the drinker's health, though real enough, must have seemed modest when compared with those posed by typhoid, tuberculosis, and smallpox.

It was not until the eighteenth century that the drinking habits of the populace first gave rise to alarm, rather than merely to the moral disapproval of preachers and clerics; and, characteristically, it was an alien drink, the Dutch spirit genever, which was responsible. William of Orange had succeeded to the throne in 1688 and had first introduced gin from Holland and then encouraged its domestic production. By the 1720s gin was being sold in the streets of London and Bristol and hawked from door to door at a penny a pint. The effects on the urban poor were devastating and plain for all to see. In 1726 the Royal College of Physicians submitted a petition to Parliament drawing attention to 'the fatal effect of the frequent use of several sorts of distilled spiritous liquors upon great numbers of both sexes, rendering them diseased, not fit for business, poor, a burthen to themselves and neighbours and too often the cause of weak, feeble and distempered children'. The petition went on to observe that the problem 'doth every year increase' and it continued to do so for another twenty-five years as Hogarth's famous engraving 'Gin Lane' so vividly portrayed. Eventually, however, in 1751, Parliament passed an act 'for more effectually restraining the retailing of distilled spirituous liquors', followed within twelve months by the Disorderly Houses Act. The result was a rapid decline in consumption.

In the nineteenth century, however, consumption began to rise again, particularly in the rapidly enlarging industrial towns, a tribute partly to the country's rising prosperity and partly to the deprived conditions in which the urban workforce was forced to live. Despite restrictions on the opening hours of alehouses (1828) and restricting the sale of beer to 'licensed premises' (1830), consumption of beer and spirits rose steadily. Wine consumption also increased sharply after the Cobden Treaty of 1860 reduced the duty on French wines. Beer consumption was boosted further in 1880 by Gladstone's free mash tun system, for this allowed brewers to use carbohydrate sources other than malt and so lowered the price. Towards the end of the nineteenth century consumption had risen to the equivalent of nearly 11 litres of pure alcohol a year for every man, woman, and child, and over 40 per cent of all exchequer funds were derived from the excise duty on alcoholic beverages.

After 1900 consumption started to fall, slowly at first but very rapidly during the First World War (see Table 7, p. 107), partly because of the controls imposed by Lloyd George's government in its determination to curb drunkenness in munitions factories. The number of licensed premises and their opening hours were both reduced, restrictions were placed on the producton of beer and spirits, their alcohol content was lowered, and it was made illegal to sell liquor on credit. Their measures appeared to be effective; beer consumption fell by 63 per cent and spirits consumption by 52 per cent between 1914 and 1918. After the war and the partial withdrawal of these controls consumption started to rise again, but it fell once more during the prolonged economic depression of the 1930s and remained at a comparatively low level until the late 1950s. Over the next twenty-five years, however, per capita consumption rose steadily, virtually doubling between 1959 and 1979. Since then there has been a slight fall, though in the last two years the trend has been upwards once more.

It is clear, therefore, that there is nothing fixed or immutable about British drinking habits. On several occasions in the last three hundred years consumption levels have changed very substantially, sometimes increasing and sometimes decreasing. There have been even more dramatic changes in the consumption of individual beverages, particularly wines and spirits. The main causes of these changes have been economic, and changes in per capita consumption usually mirror global changes in economic activity and general prosperity. As a London policeman observed in the 1880s, 'a great amount of drunkenness is a sure sign of work being plentiful'. Rising consumption in the latter half of the nineteenth century, and again in the 1960s and 1970s, coincided with periods of steadily increasing national prosperity, and the low consumption levels of the 1930s and the modest fall in consumption that occurred between 1979 and 1982 were associated with periods of economic recession.

But consumption levels are not determined purely by economic factors. Public attitudes and the legal framework which these generate also play an important role, and have often changed from one generation to the next. What tends to happen is that the cyclical changes generated by periodic fluctuations in economic activity are amplified by cyclical changes in public attitudes provoked by increases or decreases in the incidence of drunkenness and other undesirable and publicly visible consequences of drinking. As consumption rose during the nineteenth century public drunkenness and other ill effects of alcohol on public order, family life, and health became increasingly obtrusive. This generated widespread public concern and increasingly powerful temperance movements, particularly in the non-conformist churches. In North America and Scandinavia this culminated in the total prohibition policies of the 1920s. In Britain it enabled Lloyd George's government to introduce the stringent controls which reduced consumption so sharply during the First World War. As consumption fell, however, the ill effects rapidly became less conspicuous. As a result, by the 1950s a new generation had grown up with no personal experience of the evils their parents and grandparents had witnessed. They therefore had a much more relaxed attitude to alcohol. The temperance movement faded away, the proportion of teetotallers in the population fell steadily and many of the controls imposed a generation before were repealed or simply fell into disuse. Bottles of gin and handy six-packs of beer appeared on the shelves of supermarkets, the opening hours of public houses were extended, off-licences blossomed in every high street and the police turned an increasingly blind eye to underage drinking. The effects of rising prosperity were therefore magnified and consumption rose year by year. Eventually, in the mid-1970s, the point was reached at which public concern with the ill effects of alcohol began to reassert itself once more. The recommendations of the 1972 Erroll Committee for a further relaxation of English and Welsh licensing laws were ignored, the Health Education Council and the Scottish Health Education Group started trying to persuade people to drink less, James Callaghan's administration commissioned a confidential report on United Kingdom alcohol policies (the 1979 'Think Tank' Report), the World Health Organisation declared that the harmful effects of alcohol were 'one of the world's major public health problems', and the Royal College of Psychiatrists published its 1979 report, *Alcohol and Alcoholism*.

Social scientists sometimes refer to these cyclical changes in per capita consumption and the changes in public attitudes which accompany them as the 'long waves' of alcohol consumption. They are an important historical and social fact. But, of course, history never repeats itself exactly. The lessons of the past will not tell us what will follow the uneasy stalemate of the last five years: by themselves they will not determine whether the end of the recession will be followed by a further rise in consumption, fuelled by imports of cheap wine from our Common Market neighbours; or whether on the other hand an increasing concern with a healthy life-style and increasing awareness of the carnage wrought by drunken football fans and car drivers will lead to a tightening of legal restraints and slowly falling consumption.

3

Present perspectives on alcohol misuse

Thirty years ago in this country, alcohol dependence was largely regarded either as a music hall joke or as a disgrace. It was seen as something which did not have much to do with our own century, and a condition from which the British were, by grace of national temperament, deemed to be immune. The indifference of the general public was matched by lack of interest among the professions: medical schools taught only about the physical complications of advanced alcohol abuse; the NHS made no special provisions for treatment; and there was no special nursing or social work interest. Government departments saw no need for action. The nation's drinking problems were passively ignored or purposely denied.

From such neglect, over a comparatively short time alcohol misuse has become news (albeit with the story often rather muddled). To point to this change in no way implies the complacent assumption that the days of denial and evasion are totally over. The growth of British efforts and awareness has taken place within the context of wider, international changes. From the 1950s onwards, the World Health Organisation has urged that drinking problems should receive governmental attention. Expert opinion in Britain was beneficially influenced by work carried out in many other countries.

The larger part of this chapter seeks to outline the advances of the last thirty years, while the final section deals with some present dilemmas and confusions which are still seen to be in need of clarification. Developments have been evident in the provision of statutory and voluntary services and our attitudes and responses to drunkenness offences and homeless problem drinkers. The new awareness has created a need for improved education both for the public and professions; a need which has been met only partially.

Organizations have been created to provide a community and national response but they have proved of varied effectiveness. Research has shifted slowly out of the doldrums but it is very far from advancing rapidly ahead. The reason for charting both the achievements and the dilemmas is to portray the state of current awareness that has arisen out of the attitudes and historical trends described in the previous chapter. Without this it is difficult to understand at all fully the exact nature of society's extraordinarily complex responses to, and attitudes towards, its drinking and its drinking problems. Without such understanding, it would be impossible sensibly to plot any course for the future.

NEW HELP FOR THE INDIVIDUAL

Developments within the National Health Service

In most parts of the country, if a patient who was dependent on alcohol had attended his or her GP in 1950, the family doctor would probably not have felt personally competent to undertake treatment, and there would have been a stark lack of treatment facilities to which to refer for specialist help. There were a few exceptions, but most often an alcohol-dependent person would have had to take their chances in terms of an admission to a general ward of a mental hospital, where they would frequently have been far from welcome and might have found their condition little understood. A significant development took place when, in the early 1950s, the first specialized National Health Service (NHS) alcoholism treatment unit in England was established, at Warlingham Park Hospital near Croydon, Surrey. The work of this unit helped to win the NHS over to the belief that alcoholism treatment was one of its legitimate responsibilities. In the early 1960s the first Scottish unit was set up in Edinburgh and in Wales a unit opened in Cardiff. In 1962 a circular was issued by the Ministry of Health which recommended the setting up of a specialized treatment unit in each region. To date, twenty-nine such units have come into operation. Medical work on alcohol-related problems has by no means been limited to the specialized units although they continue to have a major role as advocates for improved services. In recent years specialist services have devoted more time to community based and out-patient work. With improved liaison between agencies they have at best become one aspect of a network of services meeting the needs of a range of problem drinkers.

The homeless inebriate

The problem of the homeless problem drinker has been a traditional concern of the Salvation Army and the churches, and of voluntary organizations in general. But until recently, the chronic inebriate lying out on a derelict site or the drunk begging at the street corner would often have been regarded more as a public nuisance than as a sick person deserving help. He would appear repeatedly before a magistrate for sentencing and, when not sleeping rough, circulate between doss-house and prison. He was a symbolic figure of society's uncaringness and denial – an ugly embarrassment rather than a human being. Even some of those who began to take a medical interest in alcohol problems tended perhaps at first to see him as 'a drunk' rather than 'someone with alcohol dependence', and disdained him as someone who would reinforce the worst stereotypes that gave alcoholism a bad name. In 1961, St Luke's House in Lambeth was set up as a hostel for problem drinkers by the West London Mission and provided a prototype for the specialized rehabilitation centre. Other hostel experiments soon followed, with Rathcoole House (in Clapham) providing an early example of work with drinkers who were ex-offenders. Since these pioneer efforts, other voluntary organizations such as Turning Point have developed similar houses in a large number of urban areas. An important impetus in funding such projects was the Department of Health and Social Security (DHSS) Initiative (1973) on Community Services for Alcoholics.

Therapeutic hostels

At present there are seventy-five therapeutic hostels in England and Wales which have been established by predominantly voluntary bodies and by some (albeit regrettably few) social service departments, for example in Edinburgh and Manchester. Residents need not be homeless to qualify for a place. These houses aim to foster therapeutic change rather than just offering shelter. They use a variety of group and behavioural techniques and enable individuals to spend a considerable time, usually in a 'dry' environment, rebuilding their lives. Many projects have, in addition, flatlet schemes where individuals can live for longer periods while maintaining contact with the agency and some may require permanent residence and support. A small survey for the Turning Point organization found that many people who passed through such houses did rebuild their lives successfully.

It is notable that Britain, unlike some countries such as Sweden, has virtually no long-term sheltered housing for those who are brain-damaged from alcohol.

Decriminalization of the drunkenness offence

The Home Office Committee on the Treatment of the Chronic Drunkenness Offender Within the Penal System reported in 1971 and recommended that a system of care and rehabilitation should be substituted for the traditional penal approach. It proposed the setting up of detoxification centres to which the inebriate would be taken, rather than having him locked up in the police cell. The report also proposed expansion in specialized hostels, 'shop-front' counselling centres, and other social work facilities. That a government committee could report in this way must again be seen in terms of symbolic significance as well as substance: society was declaring that alcohol-related problems were society's business, and that old evasions and denials of responsibility could no longer serve. There have, however, been great delays in seeing the report's recommendations implemented. Responsibility for implementing those recommendations now lies largely with the DHSS and local authorities, working in conjunction with voluntary organizations.

Following the 1971 report, the DHSS commissioned two experimental centres. In Leeds the centre was unconnected with the hospital service, in contrast to the Manchester hospital unit. Alternative types of facilities to which drunken offenders could be taken were also studied. These included those already providing or potentially providing detoxification services, including Salvation Army hostels, detoxification beds on a general psychiatric ward, and detoxification beds on the wards of an Alcoholism Treatment Unit primarily involved in longer-term rehabilitation.

An evaluation of five different forms of detoxification service has been published recently. This provides further support for the view that persons who have committed more than two drunkenness offences are very likely to have a serious drink problem. The damage to their health, however, may be less severe than that observed in detoxification centres such as exist in Oxford where the clientele is predominantly home-based rather than homeless. There is obviously great diversity both with respect to the needs of the clients and the services provided. Certain key functions which are required of a detoxification service were identified as: accessibility, a treatment and rehabilitation programme which could respond to a range of needs, a degree of specialization among staff, and continuity of after care within a network of community services. Studies of police referrals to a hospital detoxification centre showed that such a centre served two useful functions. Approximately a quarter of those patients who went through the centre considerably improved their social functioning and the centre also diverted potential patients away from other hospital beds where they would have been admitted for detoxification and also reduced the demands on general practitioners' services. A detoxification and rehabilitation hostel in Aberdeen has proved effective in virtually eliminating drunkenness offenders from the court.

Recently suggested alternatives include the use of low-cost sobering-up centres, where individuals can be removed from the community, briefly sobered-up, and returned (with the opportunity for further treatment subsequently) without the lengthy medical, psychological, and social assessment carried out in the detoxification centres. The latest Government initiative has been the idea of police cautioning procedures, whereby offenders are arrested, kept in police cells until they have sobered up, and then cautioned and sent on their way rather than prosecuted. This procedure, while saving some police and court time, does nothing in terms of rehabilitation for such individuals. This is a disappointing end to the optimistic plans of the 1970s: the drunk in the street is considerably worse off in many areas than he was when the 1971 report was written.

THE GROWTH OF SELF-HELP ORGANIZATIONS

Among other influences contributing to new awareness has been Alcoholics Anonymous (AA). Despite the anonymity of its individual members, AA has captured public interest and sympathy. The simple message that 'alcoholism' is an illness, and the optimistic declaration that this illness could be 'arrested', helped to overcome the popular stereotypes and pessimism. Community surveys have shown that more than half of the people interviewed named AA as a prime source of help for people with drinking problems. In this country, psychiatric hospitals and Alcoholics Anonymous have worked in fruitful partnership, with much two-way referral.

With over 1,000 groups in Great Britain, and a growth rate of approximately 15 per cent per year, Alcoholics Anonymous has ensured that in every city and in most towns a problem drinker can turn to the telephone book and make contact with help, probably within the hour. In addition to the immediacy of help, AA provides a continuity of support which so many people find invaluable. A recent national survey showed that most members go to an average of two meetings per week and are involved in a whole range of both formal and informal AA activities. One of the spin-offs from AA is that this fellowship has provided the model for many self-help organizations which now attempt to aid people who are perplexed by other types of personal problem. Al-Anon (the organization for family members and friends of alcoholics) has been important in providing help for families and developing an awareness that alcoholism is often a family problem. Al-Ateen offers support to the teenage children of alcoholics.

In the last few years another self-help group called Drinkwatchers has gradually developed. This is aimed at people who are concerned about their drinking but whose problems have not advanced to a state of severe dependence. Members learn techniques for moderating their drinking and develop new skills and interests which do not involve alcohol. Its techniques and philosophy owe much to the ideas of behavioural psychology which have had great influence recently on many aspects of the treatment of alcohol problems. The efficacy of Drinkwatchers has not yet been fully evaluated, however.

BUILDING THE COMMUNITY'S OWN AWARENESS

The specialist treatment units and AA promoted a solution in terms of treating individuals who were already more-or-less extreme casualties. This emphasis on specialist care allowed the community to avoid facing its own responsibilities – the problem was simply a few ill people who could be left to the specialist agencies. The incomplete and unsatisfactory nature of this approach has become evident in recent years and more emphasis is now being placed on giving advice about minimizing harm due to drinking at as early a stage as possible. This has meant bringing the necessary skills into the front line among social workers, general practitioners, clinical psychologists, and nurses who encounter the problem drinker at an early stage in his or her history. In some areas the specialist resources have pooled their expertise to form a community alcohol team which regards its first duty as the provision of consultation and support to the 'front line' agencies. The events which, purposely or accidentally, have moved the community itself towards greater awareness will be considered next.

In 1961, the first moves were made to set up a local Council on Alcoholism in a London Borough, and in 1962 the National Council on Alcoholism came into being as a voluntary organization dedicated to fostering the setting up of local Councils across the country. The work of that national body in England and Wales has now been absorbed within the responsibilities of Alcohol Concern.

This body was created in 1983 in England and Wales, as a result of an enquiry by the DHSS Policy Strategy Unit into the voluntary bodies which were concerned with alcohol problems at that time. It drew a number of functions within one organization. The main activities of Alcohol Concern are providing support to existing local voluntary services, most notably councils on alcoholism, organizing training courses, and the promotion of prevention.

There are approximately forty-five Councils on Alcoholism in England and Wales and twenty-five in Scotland (under the auspices of The Scottish Council on Alcohol). The 1973 DHSS Circular on Community Services for Alcoholism was extremely important in funding new councils. Recently, initiatives for the creation of local councils within England and Wales have been further strengthened by additional funding from DHSS. In part, these councils have simply contributed another element to the spectrum of available help for the individual, and the Alcoholism Information Centres which they run have provided help for problem drinkers and their families. The councils have also taken considerable responsibility for education within the community, for meeting the special problems of alcohol misuse in industry, for running courses and seminars, and for urging the better provision of help and providing a co-ordinating function in relation to treatment agencies. Their activity can mean that a community realizes and meets some of its own responsibilities. Rotary knows where to find a speaker; the mayor is the Council's vice-president; the local newspaper takes a sympathetic interest; the problem drinker is no longer quite so disdained; money is found for a hostel and the local MP asks a useful question in Parliament.

EDUCATING THE PROFESSIONALS

Another change has been better professional education about alcohol problems, although the extent to which the situation has been remedied should not be exaggerated. The Medical Council on Alcoholism, set up in 1967, has been concerned with the development of medical education on alcohol-related problems. For instance, one-day seminars are held annually in London and Edinburgh for medical students and nurses from around the country, handbooks for nurses and medical students have been prepared and distributed, and medical conferences have been organized. Taken singly, such activities and events may sound no more exciting than a listing in an annual report, but taken together they represent one example of the way in which changes in professional attitudes are slowly being brought about, and professional ignorance and indifference diminished.

In 1980, the Education Committee of the General Medical Council

(GMC) updated its recommendations on basic medical education to include the demand that students must be introduced to a knowledge of the problems which may result from the abuse of alcohol and suggested that the teaching of preventive and community medicine might include instruction in the social as well as the medical consequences of such abuse. In 1984, a medical subcommittee of Alcohol Concern (see below) was established with representatives from most of the Royal Colleges (although not the College of Surgeons), the British Medical Association, and other bodies involved in medical education, with a remit to extend and develop awareness of alcohol abuse among undergraduate students, postgraduate doctors, and their teachers.

The education of other professional groups such as nurses, social workers, probation officers, and prison officers was originally carried out by the Alcohol Education Centre, with its excellent summer schools. This organization has now disappeared and its educational activities have been absorbed by a new national agency, Alcohol Concern. The pattern of future education activities is not clear at present. It seems likely that an emphasis will be placed on the promotion of training on a regional basis.

More specialized training in alcohol-related problems is being provided in courses organized at the University of Kent in Canterbury and courses are also available at the Alcohol Studies Centre at Paisley in Scotland. As awareness of the importance of alcohol problems increases each professional group should be expected to given prominence to alcohol problems in its own curricula in both undergraduate and post-qualifying courses. The nursing profession, for instance, has recently established a number of post-qualifying courses in drug and alcohol problems.

The liquor licensing reports as stimulus to debate

Debate on the health implications of alcohol consumption has also been stirred up by two important government reports on liquor licensing – the Erroll Report for England and Wales issued in 1972, and the Clayson Report for Scotland, published in 1973. Government interference with its citizens' drinking, in terms of liquor taxation, the licensing of premises, 'permitted hours', and so on, has a venerable history. The motives behind these government measures have been various. Taxation has traditionally been the Chancellor's business, a weapon wielded in terms of budgetary rather than health interests. Licensing, on the other hand, has its origins in official concern for public order, not public health. The general shape of the present licensing laws still owes much to acute anxiety in the period 1914–18 about the impact of drunkenness on the war effort. That the Government should in the 1970s have set up committees on licensing both for England and Wales, and for Scotland, did not signal some new official awareness of the health implications of drinking; the exercises were intended to do no more than meet the routine periodic need for tidying up enactments which had grown piecemeal over the years. Both committees recommended relaxation in controls. In the event, what was to be historically important about these committees was the unforeseen vigour of medical reaction to their recommendations. Both the *British Medical Journal* and the *Lancet* produced editorials attacking proposals which they regarded as contrary to the interests of health. The relationship between drinking patterns and the country's experience of alcohol-related casualties was accidentally but unequivocally put into the arena of debate.

The relaxation of licensing laws which was introduced into Scotland in 1976 was welcomed by many sectors of the community and many believe that it has been associated with a decline in various measures of alcohol-related harm. Critics have attributed the recent improvements in Scottish statistics to economic changes and have criticized the liberalization of licensing as likely to contribute to greater availability and consumption in the future. The benefits have certainly not been as clear cut as is sometimes maintained by traders who are seeking to make alcohol even more readily available. The Scottish experience is being quoted by some as giving a lead in liberalization which England and Wales may now follow. The evidence of history, for instance the experiences discussed in Chapter 2, suggest that great care should be taken before increasing the general availability of alcohol.

Drunken driving as everybody's business

In the context of community awareness, the particular importance of the drunken driving issue was that it began to raise questions, not about the clinically recognizable 'alcoholic' or the 'skid row' drunk, but about the social implications of the ordinary citizen's own drinking. In this instance it was not the professional who had to be educated on how to treat the problem drinker but the citizen who drove a car who had to be taught about the implications of his or her personal drinking behaviour. Drunken driving was of vital importance as an example of an issue which forced an awareness that the nation's drinking problems were not all generated by a small minority of 'alcoholics' for doctors to deal with while the rest of us remained happily uninvolved.

The Road Safety Act of 1967 introduced the use of the breathalyser but proposals for random breath-testing were then and have remained unacceptable to Parliament. Increasing public awareness of the seriousness of the hazards caused by drunk driving is, however, indicated by polls conducted by the Automobile Association on the acceptability of random breath-testing. In 1968, 25 per cent of the sample polled were in favour of random testing, and 68 per cent against such testing. By 1975 the balance of public opinion had swung the other way – 48 per cent were in favour, and 37 per cent against. The Blennerhasset Report on Drunken Driving, issued in 1976, proposed a general tightening of legislation and received a favourable press. The 1980s have also seen recommendations for strict measures against repeatedly drunken drivers, both to keep them off the roads and to encourage them to seek help. (The drunken driving issue in its wider aspects is dealt with more fully in a later chapter, see p. 81.)

Public education

Two government backed bodies, the Health Education Council and the Scottish Health Education Group, have played a major role in public education about alcohol-related problems and sensible drinking. The Health Education Council has produced a series of useful booklets and pamphlets about normal and abnormal drinking. Its *That's the Limit* booklet, for example, is a highly readable and relevant summary of the important facts about alcohol use and abuse which everyone should know.

The Scottish Health Education Group has recently produced a self-help manual, *So you want to cut down your drinking*. This has been mailed on request to members of the general public and provides guidelines for changing drinking habits and monitoring consumption. Although freely available to anyone who cared to request a copy it was specifically addressed to drinkers who were concerned that they were drinking too much. A somewhat similar strategy has been adopted to the DRAMS (Drinking Reasonably and Moderately with Self-control) project. Here general practitioners have been encouraged to identify patients who are drinking in a hazardous way and to give them a self-help manual which can then be used in conjunction with regular progress checks provided by the doctors themselves. The self-help manual has been evaluated in a carefully controlled trial and the results of the study suggest that this approach was significantly more effective than more general advice.

Impact of the mass media

Whatever the activities of professionals, of councils or committees, of government departments or international agencies, their total impact on the awareness of the man and woman in the street would have had little effect if it had not been for the fact that, at some point during the last ten years or so, drinking and drinking problems became newsworthy. The daily press has carried news reports and feature articles, Sunday supplements have devoted space to alcohol problems, women's magazines discuss problems of drinking among women or the dilemmas of living with someone who misuses alcohol, and radio and television have on many occasions produced programmes on alcoholism and alcohol-related problems, occasionally trivial or over-sensational, but more often serious and informative.

The extent to which the mass media can, inadvertently or deliberately, reinforce certain stereotypes of alcohol use and misuse is a controversial one requiring much more thorough attention than it has hitherto received. It is a reassuring development to note that a significant number of journalists and producers are independently examining the extent to which assumptions about alcohol – for example, its portrayal as a mark of social status, sexual attractiveness, or personal achievement – are reinforced by factual and fictional material. While the area is too complex to permit simple generalizations and conclusions, it is likewise too important to be neglected. For some years, there was a tendency to portray drinking problems in terms of the fully dependent, usually physically and psychologically damaged addict with no clear indication that this represented the final stage of a process whose beginnings lie in the commonplace social drinking of the 'man in the street'. The past decade has seen several factual series exploring the relationship between such factors as availability, price and advertising of alcohol, and the prevalence of alcohol problems in our society, as well as providing much needed information about 'safe levels' of drinking. These are welcome signs that the portrayal of alcohol problems in the mass media is becoming more sophisticated and signs too that journalists and those working in television and radio are beginning to recognize the impact of drinking problems within their own professions.

The portrayal of drinking occasions in soap opera or other fictional programmes on TV takes up thirteen hours each week. This contrasts with approximately half-an-hour devoted to formal alcohol advertising. During peak viewing hours alcohol is displayed at the rate of three scenes an hour. Alcohol is a part of the scenery in fictional programmes. This exaggerates its significance in everyday life and thereby may influence viewer's expectations and attitudes towards drinking. Programme makers seem to have been able to cut down their reliance on cigarettes as a useful prop for scenes of tension or relaxation and could be usefully encouraged to adopt a similarly questioning attitude towards their portrayal of alcohol.

BACKING FOR RESEARCH

The degree to which a country is willing to fund research into a problem is often an indication of the seriousness with which that problem is being viewed. In the 1950s research spending in Britain on alcoholism was minimal. It was only in the 1960s that the Medical Research Council (MRC) and the Ministry of Health (and later the Department of Health and Social Security), began to provide backing for research in this field. A statement in the MRC's 1976 report that alcoholism studies were considered one of the Council's priorities areas was one indication of a change in attitude. Support to projects on alcohol still only constitutes just over 0.6 per cent of the MRC's total budget. In Scotland, the Chief Scientist's office of the Scottish Home and Health Department was active in promoting research into drinking and alcoholism. On a smaller scale, the Medical Council on Alcoholism has funded a number of important projects, and provided Research Fellowships. There are now a number of research centres scattered around the country but funds for alcohol research are still seriously inadequate considering the costs of alcohol-related problems.

THE DHSS ADVISORY COMMITTEE

A symbolic stamp of official concern was the setting up in 1975 of a DHSS Advisory Committee on Alcoholism. This brought together representatives of a wide variety of professions and organizations with an interest in alcohol-related problems and civil servants from the DHSS and other government departments. The committee produced three reports – *Prevention* (1977), *The Pattern and Range of Services* (1978), and *Education and Training for Professional Staff and Voluntary Workers* (1979). These reports generated considerable debate and promoted a wider appreciation of the widespread nature of alcohol-related problems. The extent to which they have influenced subsequent policy has been modest however. In particular, government recommendations on future services are still awaited. In 1982 the government published a document entitled *Drinking Sensibly* which reflected some, but by no means all, of the recommendations of the previous government's Central Policy Review Staff (the so-called

'Think Tank'). *Drinking Sensibly* proved, for instance, reluctant to specify a clear national policy on prevention, particularly proposals that would result in price rises that might prove unpopular to implement.

ACTION ON ALCOHOL ABUSE

In 1983 the Conference of Medical Royal Colleges and Faculties launched Action on Alcohol Abuse (Triple A). This body aims to increase public awareness about the damaging consequences of alcohol misuse and has established clear policies necessary for the control of alcohol-related problems. Its slogan 'Halt the Harm' made clear both its purpose and objectives. As doctors in many different specialties recognized the serious physical harm caused by drinking they felt it was important that the public and government knew of the risks involved. Triple A has developed a valuable function in drawing together expert opinion from many different backgrounds in order to formulate preventive policies. It also publishes a regular update on alcohol statistics, and Parliamentary debates and news items concerned with alcohol.

CONFUSIONS AND DILEMMAS

Here we set out a few issues which are fundamental to the debates that have been stirred up by increased interest in alcohol related problems. Later sections of the Report will return to some of these questions in greater detail.

A confusion of models

Interwoven with many other issues are the models of understanding which are employed when alcohol problems are defined, attitudes to them formed, policies designed, and actions taken. The ideas which produce the actions may not have been consciously formulated, but their importance can be illustrated by such a practical decision as whether the next person drunk in public goes to prison or to hospital, or what we say (or do not say) to the next intoxicated acquaintance leaving a party to climb into his or her car. The issue no longer lies simply in a choice between the old extremes of a 'badness' or a 'sickness' model, for a variety of models seem to be concurrently and rather inconsistently in use. Drinking, whether normal or excessive, can be seen simply as social behaviour, as something to be explained within sociological or anthropological concepts. Drinking can be seen in terms of an economic model, where alcohol is simply a commodity manufactured, marketed, and sold. An educational model is probably also in operation: drinking is learnt manners; prevention suggests the need for better education on how to drink; the treatment is in essence remedial education. Such an approach is in some ways close to a psychological model which analyses learning processes and offers behaviour therapies, but some alternative psychological approaches would explain drinking and abnormal drinking as a coping mechanism, would look for the role of alcohol in tension reduction, and make much of individual differences in personality. The psychiatric and medical models certainly borrow from many other disciplines and there is no one 'medical model': alcohol-related problems can occur as an accompaniment of neurosis or personality disorder, or overt mental illness, but it is certainly no part of the current medical approach to propose that such disorders invariably underlie excessive drinking. There is no intrinsic harm in having more than one model available, and it would be premature to insist that there is only one way to think about drinking and excessive drinking. But the confusion becomes harmful when models are only half worked out and their inferences too clumsily drawn; when competing models are inappropriately mixed together; or when people think they are operating on the same assumptions but are in fact radically misunderstanding each other. The same might be said for society's approach to many other complexities, for example in the field of criminology, but alcohol dependence shows these confusions in extreme form.

Multiple origins

The temptation has always been to look for 'the' explanation of excessive drinking. In terms of popular theorizing it is all due to slum conditions; or it is a symptom of too much affluence; or the stress of modern living provides the explanation; or alcohol misuse is due to bad homes and faulty child rearing; or it all stems from the drinker's personality; or perhaps alcoholics are born rather than made, and genetics hold the answer. It has to be realized that the causes of excessive drinking are always multiple and interactive and that any single-factor model of causation is not only wrong in theory, but in practice will lead to inappropriate responses to the individual, and to imperfect social policies.

The implications of calling alcohol a 'drug'

How can this rather frightening and perhaps derogatory label be correctly attached to a substance that most people use all their adult lives without being aware of any lure to addiction? The question receives close attention in Chapters 4 and 6.

The relationship between national consumption and overall damage

Until recently, the traditional view would have been that however much or little was drunk by the average citizen, a few people would be fated to become alcoholics, without the general level of the country's drinking having any bearing on the unhappy fate of this fixed minority. Cheaper alcohol, and relaxed licensing hours, would add to the safe pleasures of the ordinary drinker but would not add to the sum of casualties. However, the sharp distinction involved here between the determinants of ordinary drinking and harmful drinking has, in recent years, been challenged by a mass of research, and central to many of the arguments of this Report is a belief that the evidence shows conclusively that a country's level of drinking is the major determinant of that country's level of harm from drinking (Chapter 7).

The recognition of trouble in practical terms

In recent years there has been a drive to tell people that alcoholism is an illness which should be treated early, and yet listeners who hear that message on their radios may still be confused as to whether they, their children, or their spouses, really have a problem which requires outside help. Definition is not a philosophical but an eminently practical question for the worried individual, and the available guidelines may seem confused. Have I got a problem if I cannot happily do without a sherry in the evening? Is it true that I am at risk if I like to have a couple of drinks to get into the mood before going to a party? Have I really got a problem if I drink a bottle of whisky a day, given that I can almost certainly comfort myself by referring to someone who is drinking a bottle-and-a-half each day? Such queries deserve to be met, and the stance taken by this Report is quite simply that a person has a drinking problem if his or her drinking is, or soon will be, causing him or her any sort of harm or causing harm to any other person. The final chapter of this report offers some guidelines about 'sensible' levels of consumption.

IS ALCOHOL DEPENDENCE A TREATABLE CONDITION, OR IS THE OUTLOOK PRETTY HOPELESS?

There is much uncertainty as to how this question should be answered honestly, and it is one which is repeatedly asked not only by the patient and his family, but by the GP who wonders whether it is worthwhile trying to help or to refer; by the employer who wonders whether there is something more constructive to be done than sacking a drunken employee; and by the judge who would like to find a constructive alternative to punishment. The simple and quite certain answer is that people whose drinking is harming them can often be helped, but help does not always necessarily mean specialized treatment. However, it only adds to the confusion to quote, as if it were absolute, this or that percentage for 'treatment success in alcoholism': 'treatment', 'alcoholism', and 'success' are each very complicated ideas. These questions will be taken up again in Chapter 10.

These then are some of the old and new questions which now come into focus. They certainly cannot all be answered confidently and immediately, but if society rushes headlong past these difficult issues and ignores them, then confusion is likely to become even worse. The price of wine comes down, in real terms, and we know this is dangerous for the nation's health: a Minister refers beer to the Prices Commission because he thinks it is too expensive. A patient is turned away from a treatment centre because he or she is not 'a real alcoholic': the court makes treatment a condition of probation. In high places and in ordinary situations the underlying confusions in ideas express themselves time and again, leading to confusion in large and small happenings. In the final chapter of this book we make some recommendations which we believe would lead to a more coherent response to alcohol-related problems.

4

Alcohol and its immediate effects

Introduction

INTRODUCTION

What is so often left out of any discussion about alcohol problems is any consideration of the nature of alcohol itself. Society engages in widespread use of a drug with potent, varied, and complex actions, while giving hardly so much as a thought to the actual nature of that substance. Before this Report looks at the damages which can result from excessive drinking and examines their causes, a chapter will therefore be devoted to the nature of alcohol, and its short-term effects on human beings.

Many different substances are known to the chemist as alcohols, but almost all are so toxic that they are unsuitable for human consumption. The major exception is ethyl alcohol, which has the chemical formula C_2H_5OH. Pure ethyl alcohol (ethanol) is a colourless, inflammable liquid with a characteristic but weak smell and a strong burning taste. This seemingly unremarkable combination of carbon, hydrogen, and oxygen has been the basis of all commonly used intoxicating beverages since at least 6000 BC. Unless otherwise stated it is to ethyl alcohol we refer when talking about alcohol.

PRODUCTION AND THE VARIETIES OF BEVERAGE

Alcohol is produced by the action of yeast fungi, which ferment certain sugars to form carbon dioxide and ethyl alcohol. This process continues until the sugar supply is exhausted, or until the alcohol level reaches about 14 per cent by volume, at which concentration the yeast can no longer survive. The production of carbon dioxide is responsible for the 'head' on a glass of beer and the sparkle of champagne. Fermentation was the only method of producing alcohol known to primitive man, but in about 800 AD an Arab known as Jahir ibn Hayyan is said to have developed the art of distillation. This process of boiling and isolating the more volatile alcohol from the other fluids allowed the production of much more potent beverages.

Alcoholic drinks consist mainly of ethyl alcohol and water, but most also contain a variety of other substances sometimes called congeners; these include ethyl acetate, iso-amyl alcohol, various sugars, minerals, and B-group vitamins. Their concentrations range from 3 grams (g)

Table 1   *Production and content of alcoholic beverages*

group	example of specific beverages	alcohol content % v/v	production
beers	lager	3–6	brewer's wort fermented by yeast with hops as flavouring
	ales	3–6	
	stout	4–8	
table wines	still: red, white, and rosé	8–14	fermentation of crushed grapes or grape juice
	sparkling: champagne	12	second fermentation with retention of carbon dioxide
dessert and cocktail wines	sherry, port madeira, vermouth	15–20	ordinary wines plus added brandy or high-proof spirit and plant extracts as flavouring
distilled spirits	brandy	40	direct distillation of fermented grape mash
	whisky	37–40	double distillation of fermented barley or corn mash
	rum	40	distillation of fermented molasses
	gin	37–40	tasteless distillate flavoured by second distillation with berries, etc.
	vodka	37.5	distillation of grain
liqueurs	Benedictine, chartreuse kirsch	20–55	neutral spirits plus flavouring

per 100 litres of vodka to 285g per 100 litres of bourbon. In home-made beverages they are found at much higher levels (3–20 times higher). They contribute to the causes of 'hang-over' and other consequences. Juniper in gin, for instance, is a diuretic. Congeners probably do not have any other important pharmacological action, but they give the characteristic colour and flavour to different beverages, and in that sense are of great importance to the drinker.

A number of different systems are used to indicate the concentration of alcohol in various drinks, and these cause endless confusion. The most straightforward is the percentage of alcohol by volume (per cent v/v). 'Proof' scales are also widely used, particularly for revenue purposes. The notion of 'proof' originated centuries ago when, if gun-powder soaked with the beverage burnt on ignition, this was taken as 'proof' that the liquor was more than half alcohol. In the United States proof scale, one degree is equal to 0.5 per cent v/v. As if that were not sufficiently complicated, the British scale is characteristically less straightforward, with 57.15 per cent by volume being designated as 100° proof. Thus, a concentration of alcohol of 43 per cent v/v is equivalent to 86° proof on the American scale and 75° proof on the British scale.

Table 1 groups alcoholic beverages into categories and gives their strengths. Most British hotel and pub measures of spirits (between ⅙ and ¼ gill) can be deemed to contain 8–10 grams of alcohol per measure. Roughly the same amount of alcohol is present in the standard glass of sherry or port, the standard goblet of table wine, and a half-pint of 3–3.5 per cent beer or lager. This quantity is sometimes known as a 'unit of alcohol' or a 'standard drink' (see *Figure 1*).

Figure 1   *What is a unit of alcohol?*

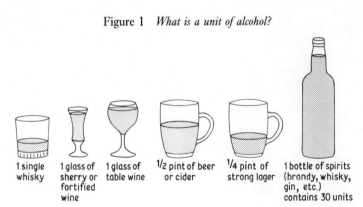

1 single whisky   1 glass of sherry or fortified wine   1 glass of table wine   ½ pint of beer or cider   ¼ pint of strong lager   1 bottle of spirits (brandy, whisky, gin, etc.) contains 30 units

Low-alcohol lagers and wines have been developed in recent years, a trend in the industry greatly to be commended. Alcohol content is kept low either by arresting the fermentation process at a very early stage, or by removing alcohol at a later stage. Lager with as low a content as 0.03 per cent v/v has been produced, though such products may contain up to 0.6 per cent v/v, and low-alcohol wines up to 3 per cent v/v.

In addition to its use as a beverage, alcohol is widely used in industry as a solvent. Industrial alcohol includes absolute alcohol (99.9 per cent v/v), and various additives which aim to make the product undrinkable. Alcohol is also a starting material for chemical products such as acetic acid, lacquers, varnishes, dyes, and artificial fibres.

ABSORPTION AND METABOLISM IN THE HUMAN BODY

The rate of absorption is influenced by a number of factors. The higher the concentration of alcohol, up to a maximum of 40 per cent by volume, the more rapid its absorption, so that absorption is slower from beers than from spirits. Other chemicals in the beverage can also be of importance: the sugars in sweet drinks retard absorption, while the carbon dioxide and biocarbonate of sparkling wines or of a gin and tonic accelerate absorption. Fast absorption gives a higher blood alcohol peak. The same amount of alcohol absorbed more slowly does not reach such a high peak but remains in the bloodstream for a longer period. Food conspicuously delays absorption of alcohol, mainly by slowing the stomach's emptying; taking a meal before a drink may reduce the peak blood alcohol level by almost 50 per cent.

Once alcohol is absorbed into the body through the stomach and the intestines, it is then distributed through the body by the blood stream. In pregnant women, alcohol, like many other drugs, crosses the placental barrier into the fetus.

In the human body, only some 2 per cent to 5 per cent of alcohol is eliminated unchanged, via the kidneys and the lungs. Although the quantity of alcohol in the air breathed out of the lungs is small, it correlates well with concentrations in the blood and tissues, and thus provides the basis for the breathalyzer test.

To give very rough guidelines (bearing in mind the considerable variation between individuals) one unit of alcohol drunk on an empty stomach will result in peak alcohol concentration of approximately 15mg per cent in a man. A given dose of alcohol produces a 25–30 per cent higher concentration in the blood in a woman than a man, even after the generally smaller body weight of the woman is taken into account. The main reason for this difference probably lies in the different body fat : water ratio of men and women. Women have a smaller body water compartment. Thus if a man drinks three pints of beer (six units) and a woman two pints of beer, they are likely to attain blood alcohol concentrations above the present legal limit for driving of 80 mg per cent. The blood alcohol concentration will fall by about 15mg per cent per hour, mainly due to metabolism by the liver. This rate of metabolism means that someone who drinks, for example, eight pints of beer at a party in the evening will still have a significant and hazardous blood alcohol level when going to work the next morning. The rate of metabolism can increase when large amounts of alcohol are drunk, and regular heavy drinkers usually metabolize alcohol rather more rapidly than light drinkers.

SHORT-TERM DRUG ACTIONS

The metabolism of alcohol yields calories, and alcohol can thus be considered a food. The calorie content is in fact quite high (Table 2) as evidenced by the 'beer belly' of many excessive drinkers. However, it is generally consumed not for its calorie content but because it changes the drinker's mood and thinking. A drug has been defined by The World Health Organisation as 'Any substance that, when taken into the living organism, may modify one or more of its functions'. Substances that alter an individual's psychological state are known as psychotropic drugs. To describe alcohol simply as a food would be to

Table 2   *Calorie value of alcoholic drinks*

quantity	beverage	calories
½ pint	beer	80
	cider	100–120
	lager	120
	stout	210
single measure	brandy	75
	gin	55
	whisky	58
small glass	sherry	65–75
	port	165
	wine	60–75

ignore its more important effects, namely its properties as a drug which affects mental functions. The remainder of this chapter will be devoted to describing its pharmacological (drug) effects, in particular its effects on the central nervous system.

General effects

When alcohol is consumed, it exerts minor effects on the circulation of the blood. Moderate doses cause a small, transient increase in heart rate. Although not a general dilator of arteries, and therefore without benefit to those with coronary artery disease, it dilates blood vessels in the skin and hence produces its characteristic flush. The flush causes a feeling of warmth, but heat loss from increased sweating may lead to a fall in body temperature. With large doses the temperature-regulating mechanism in the brain itself becomes depressed, and the fall in body temperature may become pronounced. Brandy is therefore far from being a sensible remedy for exposure to cold as popularly imagined and is in fact dangerous.

Alcohol is inadvisable for those with stomach or duodenal ulcers partly because alcoholic drinks, particularly those of 40 per cent concentration and over, cause inflammation of the stomach lining, and also because it is an effective stimulus to the production of gastric juices and acids which make the ulcer worse.

The large volume of fluid ordinarily ingested with alcohol is the main cause of increased urine flow, but alcohol also directly affects physiological mechanisms controlling production of urine.

Because of its relatively rapid evaporation at body temperatures, alcohol applied externally causes cooling of the skin. Direct application of high concentrations can slightly injure body cells, and hence the stinging sensation on the lining of the mouth caused by spirits. Alcohol also possesses a valuable local antiseptic action, but this occurs optimally at concentrations much higher than those of alcoholic drinks.

ALCOHOL AND THE BRAIN – SHORT-TERM ACTIONS

The effect of alcohol on the functioning of the nervous system is, of course, the main reason for its widespread consumption. The brain is more affected by alcohol than any other system in the body. While the exact mechanisms of the action of alcohol remain controversial, we do know that its effects are dependent on dosage and on the rate of rise in blood alcohol concentration. The first consistent changes in mood and behaviour appear at blood levels of about 50mg per cent, at which level the majority of individuals feel carefree and released from many of their ordinary anxieties and inhibitions. As the blood alcohol rises, progressively more functions of the brain are affected. Driving skill is affected at 30mg per cent and seriously affected by 80mg per cent. Clumsiness and impaired emotional judgement follow at a level of 100mg per cent, and at 200mg per cent those parts of the brain which control movement and emotional behaviour are obviously impaired. At a concentration of 300mg per cent, 90 per cent of individuals are very grossly intoxicated. Confusion and then 'passing out' and progressive stupor follow. The fatal concentration lies between 500mg per cent and 800mg per cent. The response of individuals at different doses varies a lot and inexperienced drinkers may die from a dosage which would not cause unconsciousness in the more habitual drinker. For example, a seventeen-year-old girl recently participated in a drinking contest. She drank a bottle of whisky, lapsed into unconsciousness and died.

Regular drinkers become tolerant, to a degree, to the brain effects of alcohol which in part accounts for the variation between individuals in the levels of blood-alcohol at which intoxication and death occur.

Effects on mood and behaviour

There is a school which would have us believe that alcohol in moderation is one of the safest, most respected, and most efficacious drugs in the pharmacopoea, a point lyrically attested to by Krout, an eighteenth-century American from New England who said that alcohol not only relieved the sorrowing and the distressed, but 'gave courage to the soldier, endurance to the traveller, foresight to the statesman and inspiration to the preacher ... by it [are] lighted the fires of revelry and devotion'.

Even the most casual drinker is familiar with the feelings of warmth, the heightened perception, and the relief from anxiety and stress that alcohol, in reasonable amounts, can endow. Its tranquillizing effect is well-known among the elderly, the lonely, the sad and depressed, and sufferers from chronic pain. A drink or two may revive a jaded appetite, may induce sleep, and can avert discord. Giorgio Lolli, previously president of the International Centre for Psychodietetics in New York, once stated:

'Those of us who have considered only the marriages which have been wrecked by alcohol at the cocktail hour, or the fights which have been started, or the business decisions "clouded" might look also at the many marriages which may well have been saved, at the fights which may have been averted, and at the business decisions which may have been clarified by this ceremony.'

A study conducted in 1960 at the Cushing Hospital for the aged near Boston in the United States suggested that alcohol might be a specific palliative for the loneliness and anomie of old age. A cocktail hour was introduced at this hospital during which the patients were served beer, cheese, and crackers six afternoons a week. Within two months incontinence among male patients fell from 76 to 27 per cent, the number of actively mobile patients rose from 21 to 75 per cent, and the percentage of patients requiring sedation fell from 75 to zero. It is possible of course that simply stopping the medication may have produced similar beneficial effects. One unexpected side-effect of this study was that increasing numbers of the hospital staff gave up their meal breaks to join the patients at the cocktail hour. This increase in personal contact might well have been the most important factor in bringing about improvement.

Contrary to some lay person's views, alcohol is in the true sense a *depressant* of the nervous system. Stimulant properties have popularly been attributed to alcohol because individuals under its influence often become talkative, aggressive, and hyperactive. Disinhibition is a more correct term than stimulation to describe this aspect of intoxication. However, the way in which people behave and feel when drinking is greatly influenced by what they believe they should feel – which is determined by the culture – and what is taking place in the immediate environment. A culture may attribute no stimulant properties to alcohol, and only the soporific and uncoordinating actions be manifest. In another culture or subculture, alcohol may be associated with assertion and aggression and help drinkers to legitimize within themselves violent acts. In experiments, alcohol can be given in disguised form, and subjects can be misled into thinking a drink such as strong tonic water contains alcohol. This has helped disentangle the role of beliefs and expectations. In our culture, contentment, cheerfulness, greater sociability, and reduction of anxiety are the commonest effects on mood, and to an extent they result even if the subject is told his pure tonic water contains alcohol. Whether or not alcohol is actually present, the result also depends on the mood of the occasion, the personality of the drinker, whether the drinker is alone or with others, and the sex of the drinker and any companions. Convivial social settings enhance the exhilaration of drinking. After a few drinks conversation appears to sparkle, dull people seem more interesting, and feeble jokes funny.

The disinhibiting effects of alcohol may release suppressed feelings of aggression and hostility. Numerous investigations have associated intoxication with impulsive violence. Not only do people get involved in more arguments and accidents when 'under the influence' but assaults are also more frequent.

'Hangover' is the unpleasant state felt by some the morning after drinking. Tiredness, nausea, headache, dizziness, and tremulousness are common. Individuals vary in their susceptibility. Drinks with a dark colour – red wine, brandy, blended whiskies – tend to contain more congeners and cause more hangover than pale drinks – white wine, gin, vodka. However, all drinks can produce hangover, including pure alcohol diluted. Mixing drinks is not a cause. Dehydration appears to contribute to a small extent and therefore taking alcohol in diluted forms, or with ample fluid, may help to prevent some symptoms. In common with other depressant drugs, rebound over-excitability of the nervous system occurs after single large doses of alcohol. As the blood-alcohol level falls during the latter part of the night, there is restlessness and wakefulness and some of the morning hangover discomfort can be regarded as withdrawal symptoms.

As will be described later in this book some regular drinkers get into a state in which alcohol itself is the cause of increasing anxiety, depression, tension, and fearfulness as they move in and out of repeated mild withdrawal symptoms. In this present chapter we are only discussing short-term effects of alcohol.

Effect on sexual experience

Alcohol has been thought to be an aphrodisiac. While its relaxant effect and beliefs about its disinhibiting properties may allow the inhibited greater expression of their sexuality, alcohol actually diminishes sexual arousal. A large dose diminishes or even inhibits the male erection (brewer's droop) (see also p. 99).

Sensory effects, and effects on movements and co-ordination

Focusing and the ability to follow objects with the eyes are greatly impaired even by low doses of alcohol. Sharpness of vision is relatively insensitive to alcohol. However, at high doses sensitivity to certain colours, especially red, appears to decrease and the ability to discriminate between lights of different intensity is impaired. Recovery from the effect of exposure to glare is delayed. As with vision, the ability to hear sounds remains intact, but discrimination is impaired.

Even low doses reduce sensitivity to odours and taste, and diminish sensitivity to pain.

Tests of reaction time almost all show that alcohol has a detrimental effect at blood levels above 30 mg per cent, but show no consistent effects at lower concentrations. Greater complexity of a task increases alcohol's adverse effects, and speed tests requiring sustained responses to complex stimuli are most affected. The relevance to drunken driving is obvious. The experienced drinker may show less impairment in test performance on certain tasks than the naive drinker, but it would be entirely wrong to suppose that tolerance is ever more than partial and the belief that a heavy drinker can 'handle his liquor' is to a great extent a dangerous myth.

Effects on complex intellectual functions

Moderate or even small doses of alcohol may substantially impair performance on standard intellectual tests. Memory for words, fluency in their use, and the quality of word association are all impaired. When alcohol is consumed in a social setting communication becomes more disorganized, and the conventional rules of speech etiquette may be flouted. Drinkers break into their partners' conversations more frequently, and their responses show less knowledge of what their partners are talking about.

Fine tests of discrimination, or memory, and of arithmetical ability show that impairment begins at low blood-alcohol levels, although with arithmetic accuracy is affected more than speed. Interestingly, things learned while intoxicated may be recalled better during a similar state than when sober; and although high doses of alcohol undoubtedly impair ability to solve problems low doses may occasionally help solve difficult and unfamiliar problems, perhaps through a greater willingness to try unusual lines of thinking.

The more alcohol is drunk, the more judgement is lost. Unfortunately, many people under the influence of alcohol believe that their performance is normal, or even improved. Alcohol thus tends to increase risk taking. Bus drivers given several drinks were shown to be more likely to try to drive their buses through spaces that were too small. Pain, exertion, and cold enhance the ability of drinkers to 'pull themselves together' but this gives a spurious sense of recovered competence. The benefits of the traditional black coffee are unproven, and not based on any scientific evidence and for all practical purposes the rate of recovery and the rate of metabolism of alcohol cannot be artificially accelerated.

INTERACTIONS WITH OTHER DRUGS

Alcohol is a powerful pharmacological agent which may interact with other drugs. Some commonly seen drug-alcohol interactions can be predicted on the basis of the known pharmacological properties of alcohol. For example, since alcohol is a central nervous system depressant, it may potentiate the effects of sedatives including the barbiturates and minor tranquillizers such as Librium and Valium. When an overdose of sleeping tablets or tranquillizers is taken in combination with alcohol, the resulting coma may be deeper and more dangerous.

A number of drugs, including several oral anti-diabetic tablets, can inhibit the breakdown of alcohol, and cause the accumulation of excessive quantities of acetaldehyde, with resulting flushing, nausea, vomiting, headache, and falling blood pressure.

The speed of breakdown of some drugs is dependent on liver enzymes which are also involved in the metabolism of alcohol. When the two are taken together they 'compete' for the same enzymes, and the action of the drug may be increased because of its slower breakdown; thus, individuals taking the anti-coagulant Warfarin who have an acute drinking bout may precipitate bleeding. On the other hand, the consumption of large quantities of alcohol over prolonged periods can lead to these same enzymes becoming superefficient. Thus prolonged heavy drinking doubles the rate at which most anti-epileptic drugs, for instance phenytoin (Epanutin), are broken down, and may, therefore, threaten the control of epilepsy. Pharmacists are to be commended for the increasing frequency with which they place warnings about the hazards of combining alcohol with certain drugs. These warnings are important and should be complied with.

ALCOHOL AS A DRUG

To call alcohol 'a drug' may, to the ordinary drinker, seem to propose an odd and perhaps a rather unacceptable way of looking at the familiar pint of beer or glass of sherry. The word 'drug' may suggest either a substance used in medicine, or a narcotic whose misuse is associated with illegality and dependence. The plain truth is that alcohol is in fact a drug among drugs: it is closely similar in many of its actions to substances used in medicine, and it does have the potential to induce addiction. The drinker may happily continue with his or her pint or sherry, but the drinker and society need much greater awareness of the facts. Our culture is making the decision to co-exist with the use, for fun and recreation, of a drug which is as powerful and complex in its actions as many substances which are available only on prescription.

People should know about the calorie and protein value and health consequences of the food they eat, and can take an intelligent interest in their diet without spoiling the enjoyment of the next meal. We are courting danger if we excuse ourselves from an understanding of the drugs in our diet. The traditional strategy that Western society has employed to reduce its anxieties is to pretend that alcohol is not really a drug, but that it is a beverage, a pint of this or a bottle of that. The Muslim world has always known otherwise. Our society's needs and the safety of its continued co-existence with alcohol would today be better served by a wider knowledge and admission of the true facts.

5

Alcohol dependence

Before discussing alcohol dependence this chapter will first examine the general meaning of the term 'drug dependence'. Brief note will be taken of present understanding of the biological and psychological basis of dependence. The implications of dependence will then be examined, in terms both of what it means for the individual to be dependent, and for their family and society. There can be no doubt that the way in which dependence is conceived will greatly influence the way in which society responds. Are we dealing with bad behaviour, or in any real sense with illness or disease?

DRUG DEPENDENCE: THE GENERAL MEANING OF TERMS

The terms used in this field tend to be those recommended by the World Health Organisation (WHO). In 1965, the WHO suggested that the concept of dependence could usefully replace the terms 'addiction' and 'habituation'. Dependence, not specifically on alcohol but on any drug or substance, was to be defined in the following way:

> 'A state, psychic and sometimes also physical, resulting from the interaction between a living organism and a drug, characterised by behavioural and other responses that always include a compulsion to take the drug on a continuous or periodic basis in order to experience its psychic effects, and sometimes to avoid the discomfort of its absence. Tolerance may or may not be present.'

A distinction was then made between psychological and physical dependence.

Psychological dependence: 'A condition in which a drug produces a feeling of satisfaction and a psychic drive that require periodic or continuous administration of the drug to produce pleasure or to avoid discomfort.'

Physical dependence: 'An adaptive state that manifests itself by intense physical disturbance when the administration of the drug is suspended.'

There is no need here to become too embroiled with the logic and semantics which beset the attempt to maintain a strict distinction between psychological and physical dependence, and alcohol dependence as described in this chapter obviously has both physical and psychological elements.

The central message of the 1965 World Health Organisation recommendations is straightforward and useful. This message is in essence that dependence conditions should be thought of as a family of disorders. Between the syndromes produced by one substance and by another there will be certain dissimilarities, and each type of drug dependence has its individual stamp.

But there are also common elements: a reliance on the substance to produce a desired mental effect, which reaches the intensity of compulsion if the individual tries to or has to do without it; and discomfort and/or bodily disturbance for a period once intake ceases. Once a person is dependent, and whatever the drug, a habit has been established which may be extremely difficult to shed.

The major groupings of the major drug dependencies are: (1) dependence on opium-like drugs (opium, heroin, morphia, and synthetic opiates); (2) dependence on stimulant drugs (cocaine, where psychological rather than physical dependence occurs, and synthetic stimulants such as amphetamines and certain slimming pills); (3) dependence on nicotine (a major reason for the compulsiveness of tobacco smoking); and (4) dependence on depressant substances, which include sedatives, hypnotics (sleeping tablets), minor tranquillizers – e.g. diazepam (Valium) – and, of course, alcohol.

With none of the potentially dependence-inducing drugs does use of the drug inevitably lead to the development of a dependence syndrome. For instance, there are opium smokers in Thailand who smoke only an occasional pipe. Opiates generally have a high dependence liability, and the risk of moving from casual use to dependence is greater than for, say, Valium. Nicotine is very addictive – there are a very few people who smoke an occasional cigarette on a 'take it or leave it' basis.

It is the fact that so many people use alcohol without becoming

dependent which causes incredulity when it is stated that alcohol is a
true drug of dependence. In this incredulity lies a special danger: it is
exactly because alcohol has a relatively low dependence potential that it
is easy to overlook the very real risk of dependence which is involved.

THE EXPERIENCE OF BEING DEPENDENT ON ALCOHOL

Any case history would be misleading if it were taken as adequately
representing the great variety of pictures of severe alcohol dependence
which can develop, each patterned by the individual personality and by
that individual's personal and social circumstances. The extracts from
the case histories which follow should therefore be read with that
warning in mind. They are patients' accounts not of how they came to
be dependent (though the second story touches on that question), but
of what it is like to be dependent.

Three case histories

A forty-year-old male executive: 'I don't understand it. A happy
marriage, two lovely children, successful in my work, and here I am
wrecking everything. I get up in the morning feeling sick as death –
not just physically sick, but mentally sick. Retching if I try to clean
my teeth. Some mornings I'm so shaky I can hardly get downstairs.
I don't drink in the house as that would upset my wife. Recently I'll
keep a bottle in my briefcase and have a quick drink at the station.
I'll always have a drink as soon as I get to the office. Couldn't cope
without it. A big drink, and half-an-hour later that sickness has
gone. The morning cure. Then it's just regular throughout the day
– I'm thinking of drink, planning the next drink, feeling a bit sweaty
and tense and getting people out of the room if they're staying too
long and getting in the way of the next drink. I expect it adds up to a
bottle-and-a-half of whisky each day, and never much variation. I
don't get drunk. You wouldn't know I'd been drinking now, would
you? I hate what's happening, tell myself it's stupid, promise my
wife that today I'm not going to have more than a couple of drinks.
Last summer I stopped completely for the whole of August, but
when I came back from holiday I started with just the odd drink and
within ten days it was square one.'

A retired woman aged sixty-four: 'I suppose it's loneliness, having too
much time on my hands, living by myself. It's since I gave up work
four years ago that it's begun to happen. I wouldn't call it a serious
problem, but I know it's a problem and I don't want it to get worse.

I've always liked a glass of sherry now and then and kept a bottle in the house in case friends dropped round – a bottle might last months though and I'd never drink by myself. Four years ago I found myself looking at that bottle one afternoon and thinking, well, it wouldn't hurt to have just one. I can remember the occasion exactly. Now I suppose it's two bottles a day, always sherry. Sometimes a bit more, and sometimes for a few days I cut it down. It's a problem that has just crept up on me. I don't like going out with people who don't drink, and there used to be nothing I liked more than an afternoon out shopping with my sister. In the morning I don't have what you'd call a hangover. I feel sort of shaky inside and I wouldn't say my hands were too steady. I let the cat out, make a little rule with myself to have a cup of tea and listen to the news on the radio, do some tidying up, and try not to break my rule and have a drink before 10 a.m. but it's sometimes difficult to hold out. It's all so silly, I can't believe it's me.'

The successful executive prefaces the description of his dependence by saying 'I don't understand' and the retired female civil servant says 'It's all so silly'. As well as describing dependence (of two different degrees), they each describe in their own way a common element of bafflement – a feeling which may indeed be shared by any of us when faced with the picture of dependence. Yet if one takes personal accounts such as these, it is not difficult to identify the outline of a recognizable clinical condition.

The outline of the condition at an earlier stage needs also to be known more widely. The following is an account by a man who did not himself acknowledge at this time that alcohol had caused him any real problem, yet he was most definitely moderately dependent on drink and drinking (and later lost both his job and his marriage).

A twenty-eight-year-old sales representative: 'If my wife would just accept that I like a drink most evenings and not check up on me, we'd have one of the happiest marriages. Since I was moved to a travelling job, my own car, etc. she's also worried I'll lose my licence. True, I usually drink 3 pints of beer at lunch – with clients mostly, and drive to my next appointment, but I'm careful. By 5 p.m. I'm usually making another call, preferring, I admit, my drinking customers – so that's another 3 or 4 pints. Yes, I know my blood-alcohol level is by then well over 80 – it probably was after lunch. And in the evening I just like to be with the men at my local but that's the company as well as the beer. I know I'm drinking too much. I know sooner or later I could get breathalyzed. In fact I cut down last month for two weeks but it soon crept up again. To do my job I need to drink – I'm better at it if I've had a few – it gets me over my morning blues. And I just feel good at my local with a pint in my hand – at home I get so bored and restless. Besides, it's good to have a nightcap, isn't it?'

Common elements in dependence on alcohol

Primacy of drinking over other activities

'It's always nice to have a drink after work' – though a common enough statement in regular drinkers, for most it would not indicate an immutable ritual. Most could choose to miss the drink if circumstances required it. However, friends may notice that the drinker's sense of priorities is shifting: the evening drinking becomes not one choice among several, but a commitment which has replaced even other interests, that evening of badminton, for example. The office colleague always squeezes in her lunchtime drink even when it leaves her no time for her weekday shopping. But the individual will probably only notice the changes if attention is drawn to it.

Altered circumstances – a new relationship, a change of job – may alter the routine; family obligations may take precedence. If not, then there may be the seeds of future difficulties. Drinking may interfere with duties; family and friends may feel let down. Perhaps some individuals are unaware of this, or perhaps they decide they value drink more and let it take priority. Note that we are talking here of drinking, the activity, as much as alcohol the drug. Our twenty-eight-year-old sales representative was reluctant to forego the time with his friends standing round the bar, as well as the ingestion of his evening dose of alcohol.

At the extreme, the person becomes dedicated to the occupation of drinking with all other life demands a series of optional extras. Drinking for that executive had in effect become more important than family or ambition, and the clue given by the woman who gave up her shopping expeditions can provide insight into the real force of the feelings she was experiencing. Looking back on their experiences sufferers will often describe serious lapses in behaviour, dishonesty, deceptions in personal relationships, evasions of responsibility at work, or as yet undiscovered embezzlement or theft, and it will be clear that they accord drink priority although social position, home, or health are obviously suffering, Appalling disasters may occur, but drinking takes overriding precedence.

A degree of inflexibility is visible. Whereas the ordinary drinker's intake varied from day to day, week by week, the dependent drinker's *repertoire of drinking becomes narrowed*; he or she could probably describe within fairly narrow limits exactly how each day's drinking is scheduled.

Subjective awareness of compulsion to drink and difficulty controlling amount drunk

Unless individuals are concerned about their drinking, or are trying to cut down, they are unlikely to feel anything related to a craving for drink. They may scarcely perceive any need. Drinking is part of their day; they drink when they feel like it. This is especially true if the drinker lives and works among people who also drink regularly. But if such drinkers attempt to cut down they find the habit difficult to change, particularly if they have experienced symptoms such as the edgy tense feelings of the woman in our example when 10 a.m. approached. The subjective feeling of compulsion is hard to capture in words, but anyone who is a dependent cigarette smoker will be able to empathize by recalling how the tension and craving mount if he or she is deprived of a cigarette in a situation where they would normally smoke. Repeated struggles and failure lead some individuals to feel they are compelled to drink despite themselves.

Control of the amount drunk on an occasion may be impaired. Thus the first two people in our examples reported they could no longer be sure of drinking in a way they could consider reasonable once they started. This is partly why individuals reaching this point often choose abstinence rather than try to re-train their drinking practices.

Altered tolerance to alcohol

Increased tolerance is shown by the dependent person being able to sustain an alcohol intake and function with apparent effectiveness at blood-alcohol levels that would seriously affect or incapacitate the non-tolerant drinker – hence the executive's report that he 'never got drunk'. Such an acquired tolerance for alcohol is often misinterpreted by the drinker as meaning that not much can be wrong, whereas in reality exactly the opposite conclusion should be drawn. The fact that an individual can still conduct business on a daily alcohol intake that would incapacitate the ordinary drinker is not proof of some sort of special strength or immunity, but an important indicator of increasing dependence.

An apparent reversal of tolerance occurs in some individuals whose dependence is well advanced. A man who could hold prodigious quantities of drink now falls down in the street after an amount which he was previously accustomed to drinking regularly and feels he 'needs'. It may be that he has changed from being a continuous drinker to having bouts interspersed by some weeks of abstinence in which he loses his previous tolerance. Or, his brain's ability to adapt to alcohol has been lost due to alcohol-induced damage, or liver damage may have reduced his capacity to metabolize alcohol – a very serious sign.

Repeated withdrawal symptoms

The common withdrawal symptoms are 'bad nerves', shakiness, insomnia, sweatiness, and nausea, which occur after a drop in blood-alcohol level. Especially important as a withdrawal symptom is the disturbance of mood. Sufferers may be tense, jittery, on edge, feel awful, and perhaps have attacks of panic. They can be incapacitated to the extent that they dread any social interactions, because they feel so bad in themselves; perhaps this is why our sales representative felt he needed a drink to do his job. These symptoms may at an earlier stage be only mild, occur perhaps only after several days of particularly hard drinking, and not all the symptoms may be experienced. Withdrawal is most usually experienced on waking in the morning, but can occur during the day if the heavily dependent person goes too long without a drink.

If drinking is spaced out regularly through the day, with a large drink being taken late at night, the dependent drinker may wake each day with a considerable blood-alcohol level, and successfully keep himself or herself topped up so that withdrawal symptoms are kept at bay. He or she may not know that a highly unpleasant disturbance is only a few drinks away. If tranquillizers are being taken too, these may postpone withdrawal symptoms, while deepening the intensity of the brain's chemical dependence. 'Cross-addiction' to tranquillizers plus alcohol has become more common in recent years, particularly among women.

Any circumstance which suddenly leads to reduction of intake or complete abstinence may of course precipitate withdrawal symptoms – sudden admission to hospital, or arrest and imprisonment are typical circumstances in which delirium tremens (p. 90) may develop. The insomnia which many dependent drinkers complain of is often a result of their drinking rather than its cause. Alcohol late at night helps induce sleep but as the blood level falls there is a rebound of restlessness and wakefulness at perhaps 4 or 5 a.m. or earlier.

Relief or avoidance of withdrawal symptoms by further drinking

From drinking in order to feel better, dependent drinkers drink in order to avoid feeling worse. They recognize withdrawal symptoms as such: it is not only the severe morning symptoms which have to be 'cured' (a dependent person may not be able to shave or do up buttons without a drink) but if they are severely dependent they will react to mild symptoms which occur during the day if they go too long without a drink. The executive tried to get people out of his room when he began to sense these symptoms coming on, so that he could reach the bottle in his desk. It is only when we remember the shame with which many alcohol-dependent people drink and the symptom itself that we are now discussing – the avoidance of withdrawal symptoms by repeated drinking – that we can understand why these people need to hide drink in various accessible places often in much earlier stages of dependence than we credit, and in such a manner that relatives or colleagues do not realise the amount of alcohol they get through. Secrecy, deception, dissimulation about the amount of alcohol taken, and hidden supplies can be related to this necessity to stave off or minimize withdrawal symptoms.

Reinstatement after abstinence

Alcohol-dependent persons often say that abstinence is surprisingly easy to maintain. Drinkers who have been abstinent for a week or two may have no craving, and persuade themselves that they therefore cannot have any problem, so they start experimentally to drink again – and hence the story of that August holiday and 'back to square one'. But relapse into the previous degree of dependence can follow a variable course, depending to an extent on the severity of the dependence which that person had previously experienced. Severely dependent persons are likely, when drinking again, to relapse explosively, and to return to their old drinking pattern immediately or within a few days. The mildly dependent person may take weeks or months before again experiencing withdrawal, and by then probably is moving towards more serious dependence than before.

When drinking resumes after a period of deliberate resistance, the intention to drink very moderately is rather often eroded. The tendency is to drink in the same way as before: old habits re-emerge quickly. Once started they feel they must drink to get the effect they want. They may quickly become obviously intoxicated, the nervous system having temporarily got used to being without alcohol. Or, if the sense of frustration, failure, or guilt is great, there may be a mixed sensation of release and despair as caution is abandoned.

'Aren't we all dependent?'

A condition must be recognized which exists in degrees, and not only in extreme degree. It has many elements within it, rather than any one key diagnostic feature, and is subtle, variable, shaped by many factors, and conforms to no stereotype. The mistake has been made in the past of sometimes painting the picture in such extreme terms that even that executive would be doubtful as to whether it applied to him, and the sixty-four-year-old woman would immediately conclude that alcohol dependence had nothing to do with her particular story.

The question is indeed often asked whether everyone who drinks regularly is not at least in some minor degree dependent on alcohol – the person who, for instance, would feel deprived if he did not have his evening glass of sherry. In that sense we are all in fact 'dependent' for our ordinary happiness, gratification, and emotional sustenance on a whole range of substances, people, roles, and objects; we may be in this sense reliant on family and friends, on our jobs, on our motor cars, our favourite armchair and the television set, and perhaps on a glass of sherry in the evening or a couple of pints of beer every Saturday night. Some degree of 'dependence' on alcohol, if the word is used in that way, certainly comes to be the norm, and among normal drinkers there will be a wide range of sensed need for alcohol in terms both of drinking occasions and quantity drunk. Some 7 per cent of drinkers report sometimes feeling restless without a drink. Tolerance to alcohol is also a matter of degree across the whole spectrum, from the naive drinker to the executive in our example.

But let us be clear. Severe dependence on alcohol, as experienced by the most affected 1 per cent of the population, is a very abnormal state indeed. To have reached that point predicts powerfully that a succession of physical and social problems is likely to ensue, and that attempts to readjust drinking to moderate harm-free levels may well fail.

This message must not be lost in semantic confusion. The harm associated with severe dependence on drinking is clearly documented and must not be forgotten in disputes over the meaning of words such as 'alcoholism' or 'alcohol dependence syndrome'.

SCIENTIFIC UNDERSTANDING OF ALCOHOL DEPENDENCE

Scientific understanding of alcohol dependence is still incomplete, but in recent years our knowledge has certainly advanced. Why a person becomes dependent is a question which can in the first place be taken as an extension of the question of why people drink at all or drink heavily, and these issues are dealt with in Chapter 7. To develop severe dependence it is necessary for a person to engage in at least moderate to heavy drinking. Usually this has to go on for many years, but there are instances where the syndrome develops more rapidly.

Given the necessary heavy drinking, the process of dependence is then set in train by certain biological changes that take place in the central nervous system. In simple terms, what seems to happen is that a defensive response is called into play so that the ability of alcohol to depress the activity of the brain is countered. The process leads at first to increased tolerance. This type of tolerance is a necessary prelude to development of withdrawal symptoms. The processes that have countered depression of brain activity in the presence of alcohol cause a surge of excitation when alcohol is removed. The analogy might be with the door that has a person on one side pushing it, and on the other side someone holding it shut: suddenly stop holding it shut, and the countervailing pushing of the other person now sends the door flying open with great energy.

Such an account of tolerance and withdrawal is immensely oversimplified. What needs to be emphasized is that the processes involved are ultimately susceptible to laboratory analysis, and that we no longer have to regard the biological basis of the dependence syndrome as an unassailable mystery. Alcohol has numerous effects on nerve cell chemistry and on the membrane of the cell. It is only a matter of time until a mechanism at the cellular level is delineated.

Repeated experience of withdrawal and relief of withdrawal probably sets up a process of conditioning. Alcohol dependence can be seen as a form of abnormal learning. In terms of this theory, a person is presumed to learn the compulsiveness of dependent drinking. That a drink can offer avoidance of withdrawal symptoms, as well as actual relief, would theoretically be expected to provide strong additional reinforcement of the habit.

Other cues to trigger drinking are learnt by association. The tension of mild withdrawal becomes linked to the situation in which that is experienced – the office desk, facing the dishes in the kitchen – so that the object or situation now becomes a trigger to the feeling of needing a drink and drinking. The twenty-eight-year-old sales representative had firmly engrained mental links between drinking alcohol and doing his business. This cross-association can be powerful. It can be studied in the laboratory: for example, it has been shown that an animal made dependent on alcohol will develop withdrawal symptoms from alcohol more quickly if returned to an environment in which it had previously been made dependent.

The phenomenon of reinstatement is also susceptible to study. It seems that the more severe the dependence symptoms, the more severe and rapid is their return when drinking is resumed. This can also be demonstrated in animals made dependent – suggesting that it is not merely to do with despair and beliefs in the inevitability of losing control but to do with biological forces. In a recently abstinent, severely dependent drinker, even one evening's moderately heavy drinking can produce in mild form the type of physiological disturbances seen in the withdrawal syndrome proper. Again, explanations both in terms of learning and cellular disturbance will probably apply. At present, it must be admitted, our scientific understanding of this area is still provisional.

These combined biological and learning-theory explanations of dependence appear at first to be abandoning much previous thinking in terms of alcohol dependence as a neurosis, and of the emphasis which has previously been put on the symbolic and psychodynamic meaning of drinking, or on the personality of the drinker, and the influence of the environment. In fact there need be no contradictions. These factors can all be seen as contributory antecedents to the heavy drinking, which then lead to the dependence syndrome. These original factors also continue to be part of the total field even when the psychobiological syndrome of dependence has developed, and are often vitally important aspects in our understanding of the dependent person's total predicament.

NATURAL HISTORY OF SEVERE ALCOHOL DEPENDENCE

A distinction has to be made between the development of the dependence, and the sequence of personal and social consequences which stem from the condition's progress. Developments along these two lines will therefore first be considered separately, although they are most often rather intimately related. There is enormous variability between individual stories, no absolutely inexorable march of 'phases', but none the less there are certain general principles which can aid understanding and allow us to see common elements or processes in seemingly very different case histories.

The amount of alcohol that dependent drinkers consume is only a rough guide to the severity of their experience. Certainly six double measures of spirits or six pints of beer a day will commonly result in withdrawal symptoms such as insomnia, tremor, and restlessness, but lower amounts, if taken regularly and especially if spaced out, will result in the feeling of 'needing' a drink. Whether there is a sense of difficulty in cutting down at these levels will depend partly on how pressing is the reason for cutting down, and how great are the advantages of so doing.

The evolution of severe dependence

Patients often seem able to identify fairly closely a crucial period during which they passed from their own chosen pattern of excessively heavy drinking, to a pattern of drinking that was frighteningly different. This is an account given by a forty-four-year-old painter and decorator:

'I've always liked a drink, and in my job there's quite a bit of drinking goes on. I've always earned good money. It was a matter often of a session at lunchtime, and then in the evening I'd usually go down to the local but that wasn't every night. Some days nothing, but that would have been rare, and I wouldn't be too surprised if I'd been averaging eight to ten pints for a good few years. Then three years ago I went up North on this big contract job for nine months, and was living in digs, and getting home perhaps only once a month. That was when things went really bad, and for the first time in my life I was waking up with shakes. Feeling really terrible in the mornings, really rough, but the job had to be done, so it was a quarter bottle of whisky to get me going. The "hair of the dog", you hear about it, but I didn't think that was ever going to be for me. My drinking was really terrible when that job finished but when I was home again I tried to pull out of it and things were better for a week or two. But since then it's really been on top of me, out of control, just not the way it used to be.'

Someone suffering from this syndrome will often draw this immediate distinction between 'the way it used to be' and 'the way it is now', and sensitive questioning will then reveal that the transition has been marked by the emergence, one by one, of the core elements in the dependence syndrome which have been listed and discussed in the previous section.

The idea of a crucial phase of transition raises a number of questions. How much does the length of this phase vary? Is it still possible to draw back? What sort of age variation is to be seen in the onset of this phase? How are such variations to be explained?

As regards the abruptness with which 'the way it used to be' can be differentiated from 'the way it is now', there is obviously enormous variation. Some people may reject the idea as not applying at all to their own experience – what is happening to them now is perceived just as an extension of what has been happening all along. Furthermore, they may vigorously deny there is anything abnormal about their state. Such denial has many roots – they may indeed move in heavy drinking circles where their behaviour is not abnormal; or they resent comments from others that unsettle their view of themselves and might lead to their having to decide to cut down (which at this point they inwardly do not wish or know they will find hard); or their shame about their behaviour may be too painful to face. However, if questioning is directed to the essential elements of the syndrome they may none the less be able to perceive that there was in fact a transition, not necessarily in terms of quantity drunk but in terms of ability to control the drinking. Other drinkers may be able to recognize the onset of the syndrome but will describe the experience not in terms of a precipitous development but as a matter of having experienced a few symptoms, drawn back for six months or a year, gone a little bit nearer the establishment of dependence, and then after a couple more years experienced the rather rapid emergence of the syndrome.

Although severe dependence most often becomes established in middle age, it certainly can develop rapidly as early as the late teens or emerge for the first time after retirement. The reasons for the variability in the abruptness of onset and the age of occurrence are multiple. The basic drinking pattern in which the person has been engaging is certainly important: the heavier and more continuous the drinking, the sooner he or she will become dependent. The individual with a generally troubled personality may reach an advanced state of dependence more quickly than the more mature and controlled personality, and will sometimes crash through the transitional phase and establish severe dependence with surprising abruptness. Particular events or life circumstances may do much to explain the rapidity and timing – the painter's working away from home, a depressive illness, a sudden legacy, the breakdown of a marriage, working abroad where alcohol is cheap and social patterns invite heavy drinking, bereavement, a worrying period at work, or perhaps just an accumulation of life stresses. One can think both of forces which can push people more rapidly towards dependence, and barriers which may slow down the emergence of dependence.

Once established, definite dependence seems to have an impetus of its own, and to progress. For instance, a man who was having mild morning shakes regularly two years ago will probably today be having more severe shakes. There is variation but also (unless something is done about the problem) a fair measure of inevitability about the march of events: the natural tendency is for the experience to become more fixed, rather than to remit. However, instances do certainly occur in which the drinker regains control of his drinking, but such 'control' is often imperfect and therefore disappointing.

Evolution of the consequences

Turning from the natural history of dependence to the unfolding of the history of accompanying disabilities, one is dealing with very different matters. To use the term 'natural history' with its medical implications and connotations of pathological process is legitimate when discussing alcohol dependence as a psychobiological syndrome. But the spectrum of alcohol-related disabilities involves the social sphere and all manner of interactive processes, as well as the drinker's socio-economic position and personality, and all these to such an extent that individual variation makes nonsense of any generalizations based on the medical idea of a single 'pathological process'. At one extreme, the bank manager with this disorder may remain largely socially integrated until, at the age of fifty-five, his physical health gives way. His wife may have been irritated by his habit of falling asleep after dinner and found him dull company, his colleagues may have found him a little irritable and slow at his work, but as dependence has advanced social disintegration has certainly not advanced at the same pace. In contrast, an unskilled labourer who is single, a bit of a drifter, impulsive, and anxious, with only tenuous adjustment at the best of times, may develop alcohol dependence in his early thirties, and may then find that, very much in parallel, he is losing employment, is being arrested for public intoxication, serving short periods in prison, moving towards the forgiving friendship of the bottle-gang in the park, and then heading rapidly towards 'skid row' and total degradation – and with morning shakes relieved by a swig of surgical spirits. In many different ways, the manner in which society and the individual's close associates deal with the drinker will affect the development of consequences. Getting sacked, divorced, or arrested will cut the strands of the network of social supports and may lead to increased dependence which, in turn, may cause further social disapproval and isolation.

THE IMPLICATIONS OF ALCOHOL DEPENDENCE

What then are the immediate implications of alcohol being a drug with dependence-producing properties? It may be best to look at this under three different headings: the implications for the individual dependent drinker; those for his or her family; and those for society at large.

For the individual the implications are that he or she is handling a substance which is dangerous not only in direct terms of the disabilities it may inflict (Chapter 6), but dangerous also because he or she starts drinking more heavily than ever originally intended, and is not able to pull back easily at all. Once a person has become severely dependent there is often little choice between continuing to drink destructively or stopping drinking altogether. The individual needs to come to terms with the fact that an unpleasant and destructive condition has developed, and unless he or she stops drinking he or she is likely to experience some alcohol related catastrophe, or slowly and un-dramatically to ruin health and happiness. To put matters thus may seem too highly coloured, but the misery for the individual which can often result from alcohol dependence needs to be very clearly realized.

Any person who drinks should be aware that he or she is using a drug which can induce dependence, and all that needs to be done to contract this condition is to drink for long enough in sufficiently large quantities. No one has a guaranteed immunity. There are individual variations in what constitutes the danger zone for dependence risk. The levels of drink which may harm health are lower than those which induce dependence, and the important question of what constitutes 'sensible drinking' is discussed later (pp. 176–79).

The implications for the family of the alcohol-dependent individual are that unless they understand what they are dealing with, they will be apt to use the wrong tactics. The analogy might be with the mistake that would result if a man's wife tried to jolly him out of his 'indigestion', when he was in fact beginning to experience symptoms of a duodenal ulcer. Drinking, where the problem has progressed to a stage of well-established alcohol dependence, is not going to be brought back under control by any amount of cajolery, scolding, striking of temporary bargains or simply hoping that the situation will improve.

As for the implications for society, we have to acknowledge that there will be many people who are using alcohol in a way that is excessive, but whose drinking, because of the very nature of dependence, is not going to be brought back under control by ordinary disapprobations or punishments. Taking alcohol-dependent people off one's list of friends will not necessarily make them drink more reasonably, and neither in all probability will sacking them, or putting them in prison. It is this diminished responsiveness to ordinary social remedies that so often frustrates society's well-meaning efforts to deal with the condition by using methods which are largely inappropriate to the nature of that condition, and which may if anything make matters worse. The implications of alcohol being a drug of dependence have therefore to be considered not just by the families of those people, not just by the professionals responsible for treatment and the government departments responsible for organizing treatment but by everyone. The alcohol-dependent person may be our employer or employee, our burglar, our policeman, or our judge, our patient or our doctor, our father or our daughter, or ourselves.

DEPENDENCE AND THE IDEAS OF SIN AND DISEASE

In the light of what has been discussed in this chapter about the nature and significance of dependence, this is the point again to take up the questions of 'models of understanding' (pp. 7–10).

The sin model

What are the social profits and losses which follow from the sin or self-indulgence types of formulation? The immediate profit for society is that there is someone other than society to blame. The argument is that we can hardly be expected to take blame or responsibility for people who of their own unimpaired and sinful volition drink in a manner that causes them to suffer. If they fall down in the street they should be fined, and if they cannot pay the fine they should go to prison. Many of the 100,000 arrests a year for public drunkenness are of people who are not casual roisterers but, particularly among those who offend more than once, prove to be men or women severely dependent on alcohol. The sin model of excessive drinking, though not one on which any Minister of State would care publicly to take his stand, thus still dictates aspects of the way things are officially handled. It also influences or wholly dictates the dealings of many ordinary citizens with the excessive drinker with whom they come in contact: the person we sack, the person we no longer ask to dinner, the person whom in every sense we pass by on the other side of the street.

A harshness in public attitudes towards the victim might be thought to deter some people from drinking in such a manner as to contract severe dependence, but this may not in fact be effective. Society can happily condemn the advanced case of alcohol dependence while in no way disapproving the type of drinking that leads to that condition. In terms even of society's self-interests the model soon ceases to be very satisfactory. We find that punitive attitudes or legally inflicted punishments do little to deter this behaviour. Punishing the heavily-dependent person seems pragmatically as ineffective as whipping the mentally ill or imprisoning the bankrupt. The sin model is simply not a good basis for effective policies in society's interests, even disregarding its invitations to humanity.

The disease model

Not surprisingly, an alternative model has been sought, and the most important contender of recent years has been the disease concept of alcoholism – with the word 'alcoholism' used here in a manner akin to severe alcohol dependence. The statement that 'alcoholism is a disease' has at times been propagated without asking what is meant by 'disease', or by 'alcoholism'. Partly for this reason, this model has recently come in for some questioning.

Leaving aside for the moment any questions as to the scientific validity of the disease concept, it is again possible to examine the social profit and loss which comes from looking at the condition in this way. The likely immediate gains are of course evident in the kinder approach which this model should propose in our dealings with the individual – if a person is ill, we should take him or her to a hospital rather than a police cell, we should perhaps provide sick leave rather than the sack, we should seek marital therapy rather than immediate divorce, and so on.

There is, though, a danger in the disease concept if a consequence is that privileged status is then given to the subgroup of excessive drinkers who manifest dependence symptoms, while those many people who are drinking self-damagingly or harming others but who have not developed this syndrome are considered to be undeserving of help and concern. This sharp dichotomy has at times found expression in the distinction between 'the real alcoholic' and 'the drunk'. All that has been said in this chapter about the reality of dependence intentionally supports the notion that there is something special about the position of a particular and identifiable subgroup of excessive drinkers. But even the severely dependent drinker is not an automaton in the grip of an all-controlling and pathological process which totally denies his self-responsibility. At the same time the man or woman who is drinking excessively only at weekends, and who is violent or aggressive when drunk, may warrant as much sensitive and compassionate understanding as someone who has the greatest difficulty in controlling his or her impulses.

The model best suited to society's needs

Alcohol problems provide an unusually visible demonstration of the importance of society's ideas as determinants of social transactions. There is the real question as to whether the policeman or the ambulanceman picks up the drunk collapsed in the street.

Which way of looking at things can today be recommended as best suited to society's needs? What we are looking for here is not the most scientifically correct manner of defining alcohol dependence: the discussion of the psychobiological basis given earlier in this chapter should make it clear that science is at present in no position to rule dogmatically on the nature of the dependence syndrome. But the scientific evidence does strongly suggest that what alcohol-dependent people have long been telling us about their sense of compulsion, their craving, and the impaired ability to control their drinking probably has a basis in physiological and psychological processes which we are beginning to unravel. The dependent person's relationship with alcohol is not on the same footing as it was in his or her predependent, heavy-drinking days. In these terms, in our particular society and at the present time, it may be useful to regard dependence as a disease, but with the added insistence that society has to take an informed rather than a mechanical view of what is meant by that statement.

It is in accord with an informed notion of illness to see the individual as retaining much responsibility for helping him-or herself. And there is nothing in such a view that denies the importance of the social and psychological factors in the genesis of the disorder, its perpetuation, or what happens to the ill person. Neither is the individual's self-responsibility denied. Indeed, the view of alcohol dependence which we would invite is not unique: the model is one which should be the theme (with many variations) in understanding much of what we today call disease or illness, composed of biological factors but also of social labels and of concepts of self. If society is able to find a satisfactory way of looking at alcohol dependence, it may in the process have found an appropriate way of looking at much else besides.

6

Alcohol-related disabilities

This chapter reviews the types of damage which may result from excessive or inappropriate alcohol use. What we are concerned with here is the great array of minor and major problems for which alcohol can be a cause or a contributory factor. Individuals do not have to be alcohol dependent to experience harmful consequences from their drinking. This account sets out to provide a broad picture of the types of alcohol-related problems and the extent to which they occur, rather than to present any comprehensive and detailed listing.

GENERAL CONSIDERATIONS

For convenience alcohol-related problems are considered under three headings of social, psychological and physical. In reality an individual's experience may often involve a clustering of these types of difficulty. A problem drinker's marriage may deteriorate (social disability), which causes unhappiness (psychological disability). This is followed by even heavier drinking, which causes liver damage (physical disability).

What must also be emphasized is that disabilities exist in degrees, and what is particularly needed is an awareness of the minor and less dramatic forms of damage that alcohol misuse can inflict upon an individual's life.

Everyone recognizes that grossly excessive drinking can lead to the break-up of a marriage: what is not so well known is the frequency with which drinking may insidiously and rather undramatically damage a marriage. There are too many small arguments, and neither partner puts the cause down to drinking. Time in the pub becomes more important than time at home. The home is always just that little bit short of money. Too often, perhaps ten years later when the problem has progressed to the point of marital breakdown, the couple look back and realize that alcohol misuse has been eroding the happiness of their marriage for a long time.

The question of causality, the precise meaning to be given to 'related' in 'alcohol-related disabilities', needs scrutiny. It is usually false to suggest explanations in terms of single causes: the marriage did not break down simply because of the drinking, but also perhaps because of temperamental differences between two people, because of lack of satisfaction, because of unemployment or poor housing, and so on. These factors may all indeed have contributed to the drinking; the drinking then makes everything worse, and the process becomes circular. Such a perspective is important for sympathetic understanding of the individual case, and as a basis for understanding the varied types of help which may be needed.

As an illustration, here is an account given by a woman whose husband has a drinking problem:

'I'd say the first year of our marriage was all right, but then after the baby was born and we were still living with my parents and hadn't got a place of our own, well he'd go off with some of his old friends and you can't blame him. When we got a little flat, that was a bit better, but after our third kid was born I was very depressed and I think that got him down. We had rows, and I'd threaten to go back to my mum. Then he was out of work and that didn't help. I suppose looking back a lot of those rows were when he had been drinking.'

The inadequacy of attributing all of that family's problems solely to alcohol is manifest. The crudeness of that assumption is dangerous. But perhaps the more common danger lies in overlooking the subtly destructive influences of the excessive drinking: without the drinking, that young couple's marriage might have worked out happily, they might have coped more constructively with the very real stresses of their environment.

Alcohol-related problems are not uniformly distributed throughout the population. Rates of officially recorded problems, such as hospital admissions for alcohol dependence, drunkenness offences, and liver cirrhosis deaths, are generally higher in Scotland, Northern Ireland, and Northern England than they are further south. Men are more likely than women to drink heavily and accordingly experience higher rates of alcohol-related problems than women. Even so, levels of alcohol misuse among women have risen in association with the upsurge in alcohol consumption that occurred during the 1960s and 1970s. A Scottish survey by the Office of Population Censuses and Surveys indicated that alcohol consumption among women had risen substantially between 1976 and 1984, while that among men had remained virtually static. Many agencies have noted that there has been a rise in the proportion of identified problem drinkers who are women. Women generally report drinking far less than do men. Even so women often experience alcohol-related problems at lower levels of consumption than men.

The precise type of problem that may ensue from drinking depend upon the chemistry of alcohol (a depressant drug), the characteristics of the drinker, and the context of use. In the United Kingdom many alcohol-related problems are attributable not to chronic heavy drinking or alcohol dependence (although these are serious) but to intoxication.

Given the provenance of this Report, it may seem surprising that the section on social disabilities is longer than the sections either on mental or on physical disabilities. We believe indeed that social disabilities should receive wide attention. This should not be taken to imply an underrating of the profound seriousness of the many possible adverse effects of heavy drinking on mental and physical health, and those elements of disability will also be examined.

SOCIAL DISABILITIES

The idea of social disability implies the failure of the individual to perform adequately in any role expected of him or her (spouse, parent, or employee, for instance). A closely linked idea is failure to meet expected obligations – for example, to contribute to the national wealth. The concept can also comprise the notion of any behaviour which positively transgresses social rules – crime, sexual deviance, or simply 'being a problem drinker'. That social disability is highly dependent upon social norms needs to be stressed, and the judgements involved are by their nature based on social norms rather than objective facts, with society the rule-maker and referee. The rules may be different for men and women, for different age groups, occupations, between social classes, and certainly between countries. Happy and successful social adjustment is always something of a balancing act. One important aspect of the disability may be the way in which society reacts to persons who are manifesting that disability, since this may amplify the handicap – the men or women who for instance cannot get a job because they have been labelled as a 'problem drinker'.

Social disability and the family

The impact of excessive drinking on marriage was given in the introduction to this chapter as an example of the graduated nature of alcohol-related disabilities and the multiplicity of its causes. Divorce is common: a survey of Alcoholics Anonymous showed that drinking had broken up marriages in over 30 per cent of members. As for violence, in one study of 100 battered wives, 52 of the victims reported that their partners engaged in frequent heavy drinking. Excessive drinking is associated with a wide range of problems involving families and children. It is important to note that, as with many other crimes, the *involvement* of alcohol does not necessarily mean that drinking is a *cause* of these problems.

The tangible effects of profound stresses on the excessive drinker's spouse, the addition of small stresses, and the continuing uncertainty about how each day will turn out, are cumulative. Some spouses of problem drinkers may show, for a long period, an extraordinary capacity to cope and put on a bold front: they will be smartly dressed, the children will look well cared for, the house will be spick and span, and the neighbours will not know that there is anything amiss. Money problems will be met by the wife going out to work and perhaps undertaking further training.

More often the impact of stresses soon becomes obvious. Friends and neighbours when they see that wife ask her, 'What's wrong?' She is obviously a bit worn and tense. She may well start to shut herself off from social contacts just because she doesn't want to be asked this kind of question, and thus she becomes increasingly isolated. She goes to the doctor about her 'bad nerves' and, if he is not someone to whom she feels she can talk (and a person who has time to listen), her distress will simply be met with the prescription of a tranquillizer. A woman who is under such pressure may indeed develop a depressive illness, and when she comes to a psychiatric clinic this can be the first occasion on which her husband's problem comes to notice.

Sometimes the first indication may be when the wife makes a suicidal gesture as a plea for help. A recent study showed that one-third of women admitted to hospital because of a drug overdose had a complaint about their husband's drinking. The family's problem may also come to notice when the wife turns up at a casualty department with bruises or broken bones. Occasionally she will herself start drinking excessively ('if you can't beat them, join them'). More rarely a woman will, in desperation, physically assault her drinking husband, and the extreme result has on rare occasions been murder.

To discuss the impact of drinking on marriage without referring to the situation where the wife is the excessive drinker would be incomplete and inappropriate. The disruption that this can cause is often marked by a great deal of distress and confusion, and coloured by the general tendency of society to be particularly punitive and moralistic towards the woman concerned. A husband may be ashamed and angry that his wife is bringing disgrace on the family. A woman may see her drunken husband as frightening, while a husband seems often to react to a drunken wife with a revulsion that is linked to feelings learned in our culture about betrayal of the goodness and purity of womanhood. Anger may turn to violence and, for economic reasons and because of society's pressure on women as 'carers', it may be easier for a man to leave a drinking wife than the other way round.

The disabilities which affect the children of a family in which there is a drinking problem can be devastating. Children may have to endure perpetual rowing between their parents or be witness to scenes of physical violence. The drunken parent may repeatedly pick on one particular child in the family as a target for nagging and demeaning verbal attack, or actual violence.

> 'You could always tell when he'd been drinking. He'd pick on John, our second son, he's just twelve years old now. Say he was no good, wasn't a real boy. My husband was an athlete you see, and John is on the slight side, a bit weedy, wears glasses. He'd be at him again as soon as he got into the house. Go up close and shout at him. The boy would get so terrified he wouldn't be able to speak and then his father would shout at him for an answer.'

It is not only the positive traumas that can damage the child's health and emotional growth, but the negative effect of the lack of a good relationship and of a consistent model.

The immediate consequence may be that such children develop overt neurotic symptoms, or behavioural problems, or engage in delinquency. Conversely they may become superficially very well behaved and responsible, relinquishing their right to be children and entering a premature adulthood with a stunted capacity for enjoyment.

An adverse impact on school work is common. In adolescence escape may be found by spending little time in the home to which they are ashamed to invite their friends, and finding a set of friends outside. The adolescent may drift to a peer group which is itself in some way disturbed (a group for instance in which a lot of drinking or drug taking goes on). The impact can be as great on a girl as a boy, and the psychological damage done to a girl who is torn between love and hatred for a drunken and unpredictable father can be devastating. Indeed, in many instances the emotional harm done in childhood, whether to son or daughter, will result in disabilities which continue into the child's adult life. A commonplace consequence is that such children may have difficulty in forming relationships. The parental message often given to these children is 'Don't talk, don't trust, don't feel'.

Drinking problems and employment

Some occupations have exceptionally high rates of alcohol problems, such as liver cirrhosis deaths, and alcohol dependence (see p. 124). These 'high risk' jobs include the drink trade, catering, the armed forces, the merchant navy, fishing, the medical profession, and journalism. Many reasons have been identified to explain why some jobs do have such high rates of alcohol problems. These include availability of alcohol at work, separation from normal social or sexual relationships, freedom from supervision or support, strains and stresses In some cases it appears that heavy drinkers seek out employment where they believe free or cheap alcohol will be readily available.

Excessive drinking can result in sacking, repeated sacking, and then virtual unemployability. It often means a slide into less skilled and less responsible work. In a study of Alcoholics Anonymous, 63 per cent of men had at some time been sacked because of their drinking. An earlier study showed that, in a predominantly middle-class group of alcohol-dependent patients, 52 per cent had been sacked for drinking. In a survey of people attending counselling centres in England and Wales, 45 per cent were currently 'off sick' or unemployed. Of the total, 47 per cent said that their present or most recent job represented a demotion in wage terms. Forty-three per cent believed that their drinking has caused or contributed to an accident at work. There is also good evidence that those who drink excessively will be more likely than their colleagues to become unemployed during periods of recession.

However, the impact of excessive drinking on employment must be seen not only in terms of sackings, accidents, and long spells out of work, but also in more subtle processes. A man or woman is still at work, but is not working efficiently, is getting in someone else's way, or leaving someone else to do the job. The person may not be sacked, but is promoted sideways, or retired with a costly golden handshake. Drink-related problems are likely to be experienced at every level in industry and commerce, and are as often to be found in the boardroom as on the shop floor:

Anna, aged 38, was a university lecturer in social science. She had achieved a high academic reputation but developed a dependence on alcohol which became increasingly apparent at work. She failed to read students' essays on time, she frequently cancelled tutorials at the last minute because she was too hung over to attend. There had been a number of comments about her unreliability from students and staff members. Her department was aware of her difficulties and attributed them to her stressful home life with an aged mother. Her colleagues did not like to confront her about the excessive drinking which was evident from her behaviour at staff receptions and the smell of alcohol on her breath at morning staff meetings. Many of her classes and students were transferred to other members of the department and less and less was expected of her. She was seriously injured in a bicycle accident on her way to work one morning, became a permanent invalid and never returned to work. At the time of the accident her blood-alcohol was 140mg per cent.

Drinking and crime

The relationship between drinking and crime emphasizes the need to think about causal systems rather than single causes. A criminal offence is seldom committed for one isolated and simple reason – for instance, a woman steals from a shop when she is drinking, but she is also depressed and has become impulsive or wants to be caught and given help. Because she is obviously shabby and drunk and the shop employs a store detective, she is caught. To say that drinking 'caused this crime' would be an oversimplification.

The connections between crime and drinking appear to be of several types. First there is the fact that being drunk and incapable in a public place, or drunk and disorderly, constitute offences. Strictly speaking it is not the intoxication itself which is the offence, but the immediate consequences of the intoxication. The discussion on 'Skid Row' in the next section of this chapter should make it clear that, although an individual is arrested on a drinking charge, drinking may be only one facet of the problem. Drunken driving will also be given separate consideration under a later heading.

The bulk of alcohol-related crime is comprised of petty offences committed by people who are caught up in a way of life characterized by social instability – people who are unskilled, who do not stay for long in one job, who are homeless and often itinerant between cities, and who are in many ways socially and personally handicapped. The person who is prone to break society's rules in small ways is even more likely to commit some foolish and not very profitable theft when drunk, to throw a stone through a window, to beg, to assault a policeman, or to urinate on a doorstep. If they do this sort of thing often enough and cannot pay the ensuing fine, they may well find themselves in prison. Such a crime is often described as petty or minor, but it all contributes to a process which can be profoundly disruptive to an individual's life adjustment. He or she is dragged further into an entanglement from which there is no escape, and repeated short-term imprisonment only exacerbates the predicament. He or she may as an individual be a very unimportant 'criminal', but the sum total of such people makes a major contribution to the cost and work load of the courts and the population of the prisons. The story of the drinking problem is seldom seen as worth pleading in court. Different studies of prisoners in England and Scotland have suggested that half to two-thirds of the men and about 15 per cent of the women have a serious drinking problem, and most were petty recidivists. Recent British studies have indicated that heavy drinking is a frequent precursor of both violent and non-violent crimes. In addition it is widely documented that 30–50 per cent of burglaries are committed while the perpetrators are under the influence of alcohol. In some cases intoxication may predispose people to break the law; others report drinking before committing a crime in order to reduce their anxiety at the prospect. It also doubtless contributes to clumsiness, thereby increasing the chances of detection.

There is also an association between drinking and some more specific and serious types of offence. There can be no doubt that excessive drinking quite often lies behind the story of the accountant who is suddenly discovered to have defrauded his firm of thousands of pounds or the solicitor who has betrayed a client's trust, or much more often and on a less grand scale of the storeman who has been selling off his firm's goods. Drinking costs money, and that solicitor may not only have been spending £3,000 each year directly on alcohol, but drinking may in addition have led to a life-style where profligate spending was the order of the day. Excessive drinking thus certainly makes its contribution to 'white-collar crime', as well as to the problems of 'Skid Row'.

Drinking also seems to be related quite frequently to the acting out of sexual fantasies which are otherwise kept under control. Drinking may be a contributory factor to behaviour which would be out of keeping with a person's character, and which may leave him or her aghast upon awakening and realizing what has occurred.

Another connection is that between alcohol and crimes of violence. The incident may be a fight on the pavement outside the pub at closing time when a drunken man becomes cantankerous. Drunkenness is a major factor in the increasing level of violence experienced by staff in accident and emergency departments. In a recent series of 102 incidents, alcohol proved to be implicated in 71 cases.

With intoxication there is always the possibility of sudden extreme loss of impulse control, and of violence going beyond anything originally intended. A marital argument may, for instance, suddenly become brutally serious, and a knife is used. Studies of the relationship between intoxication and murder have generally shown that in about half the cases the assailant is intoxicated at the time of the killing (and murder is, of course, very largely a family crime). There is further evidence to suggest that the victim, too, will often have been drinking heavily at the time of the event.

Excessive drinking has been identified as a factor underlying football hooliganism. This led to the introduction of the Criminal Justice (Scotland) Act in November 1980, which banned the carriage and consumption of alcohol by supporters at certain sporting events, notably football matches, and on private hire coaches en route to matches. Such legislation has been widely welcomed and has proved effective. Even more thorough controls of alcohol at football matches were introduced into England and Wales in 1985 following a series of riots and disturbances in which drunkenness played a prominent part. It should be noted, however, that at the time of writing these controls are being side-stepped by clubs applying for, and getting, exemptions from prohibition of alcohol sales.

Putting together what is known of the considerable involvement of excessive drinking in the petty recidivism that crowds our prisons; the direct involvement of drinking in public drunkenness, drunk driving, financial offences, sexual offences, and crimes of violence, it becomes evident that we have here another major reason for society to be concerned about drinking. Even with cautious regard for the need to work with an idea of 'cause' which is subtle and complex rather than single-factor, it is clear that, in any debate about crime prevention, help for offenders, or costing of the national bill for crime and correction, excessive drinking is a major and recurrent theme.

To put this problem under the general heading of 'alcohol-related disabilities' might at first seem strange. Given that society foots a considerable bill, that the person at the receiving end of petty crime suffers minor loss or inconvenience, or that the occasional victim of the major alcohol-related offence is grossly harmed, it may seem too compassionate to designate the person who commits these offences as suffering from a disability. The term is, however, being used advisedly, for the person who commits such crimes is often involved in a process which is as damaging to the individual as to society:

> 'It was stupid. I just went up the front steps, into the hallway, took an alarm clock, and then I was so drunk I fell down the steps. That's what they tell me, but I don't remember anything about it. That's always what happens when I go on the drink – I go and nick something absolutely stupid, in broad daylight. The magistrate gave me a chance last time, but you can't blame him, he's fed up now.'

There is no one case which can illustrate the whole range of alcohol-related crimes. There are certainly instances where the offender appears primarily to be a career criminal, and he has developed a drinking problem rather late in the course of that career. Drink has been employed to provide Dutch courage for quite intentional crime, and one may sometimes suspect that drinking is being used as an excuse for behaviour that was soberly premeditated. But the more closely one considers the woman who steals the alarm clock, the accountant who embezzles, the man who knifes his wife in a drunken quarrel, the more one sees the common elements of behaviour that would have been unlikely to have occurred without drinking – behaviour which is characterized by lack of impulse control or is so out of character as to suggest marked impairment of personality. This kind of behaviour brings that individual little or nothing in the way of real gain or satisfaction, and has as its largest result a disability that is the destruction of that person's place in society.

'Skid Row' and the chronic drunkenness offender

In most large British cities the sight of a couple of dishevelled people sitting together in a doorway, sharing the contents of a bottle, is quite common. There may be particular street corners or parks where such individuals are especially likely to congregate, or they may make the main railway station their haunt. The great majority of such destitute people are men. Occasionally there is a woman in the group, but she is usually isolated or drinks in derelict buildings, out of the public gaze. There are 10,000 people in this country who belong to the drifting world of what is often termed 'Skid Row'. In United States cities, 'Skid Row' has been used to describe well-known and circumscribed city areas such as the Bowery in New York. The phrase catches the image of broken-down housing, an area of rooming houses and cheap hotels, streets where the doorways will be littered with empty bottles, and a population of destitutes. Many of these people will be chronically heavy drinkers, but such an area gives a home of a sort to every kind of social casualty. A close acquaintance with big cities in the United Kingdom reveals a world which in its social meaning is very similar to the United States' 'Skid Row', but instead of being concentrated and highly visible, it is diffuse and easily overlooked.

What in this country is the meaning of the 'Skid Row way of life'? In so far as most people are aware of this problem, it seems sad, unsightly, vaguely offensive, and somehow very old-fashioned that there should still be drunken vagrants on our streets. The ordinary citizen may give a few pence 'for a cup of tea', but how the man who begs from us came to be in this state, and who he is are questions which tend to remain unasked as we hurry by.

Much information has been gathered recently on the nature of this problem. Destitute people are not necessarily all heavy drinkers – they may be eccentrics, schizophrenics drifting without support, people whose multiple handicaps have somehow dragged them down, or young and unemployed. Drinking, however, makes a substantial contribution. A study of men resident on a particular census night at the Camberwell Reception Centre in London showed that 49 per cent admitted to drinking problems. The usual picture of 'Skid Row' alcohol dependence may best be interpreted as that of alcohol misuse shaped by the particular vulnerability of the person who starts with few social supports, and whose drinking then knocks away those minimal props he or she did possess.

A survey in London showed that, among a group of fifty-one 'Skid Row' drinkers, 37 per cent were Irish, and 27 per cent were Scottish. They are perhaps using the anonymity of that city as some sort of retreat or hiding place. They often come from a home which has been handicapping, and 58 per cent of men in the London 'Skid Row' study had experienced parental separation in childhood. From home they easily move to drifting and rootlessness. They have typically never been married, and have never acquired any job skills. The drinking history intertwines with all the other social handicaps. They may start to drink regularly as soon as they leave home. By the time they are thirty they have become alcohol dependent. In their early thirties an alcohol-related offence takes them for the first time, to prison. By their late thirties they are on 'Skid Row' – chronically drunk, repeatedly arrested, in and out of prison for short sentences, sleeping in derelict houses or cheap hostels, totally isolated from friends or family, and prone to accidents, chronic chest infections, and tuberculosis. They are in a situation from which it is exceedingly difficult to find any way back. They drink cheap wine, cider, or surgical spirits. Their life expectancy is greatly shortened.

'Skid Row' exemplifies certain generally important truths. It provides an instance of society's inability to live with some painful realities other than by strategies of denial and avoidance. 'Skid Row' has always been someone else's problem. It shows our ability to get caught up in absurd and unproductive responses – the man who is arrested one hundred times for public drunkenness will inevitably be dealt with in exactly the same way on the one-hundred-and-first occasion. In a study conducted some years ago in London, 150 men who appeared before two courts on drunkenness offences were interviewed. For 25 per cent of these men it was their second drunkenness arrrest within the space of one month, and 50 per cent of the total had been arrested at least once before during the previous year; 10 per cent had been arrested more than ten times during the previous year, about 50 per cent showed evidence of the fully developed alcohol dependence syndrome, and a further 25 per cent, though not manifesting this syndrome, none the less had a serious drinking problem. These individuals showed an extraordinary degree of social isolation: almost 60 per cent were homeless, over half had not had contact with parents or siblings for over a year, and 40 per cent were unemployed at the time of interview. More than half came originally from Scotland or Ireland. The problems of the chronic drunkenness offence and of 'Skid Row' largely overlap.

Table 3 presents details of recent convictions for drunkenness. These convictions were rather more commonplace in Scotland than in England and Wales until 1980. Since then the reverse has been true. Some explanation for this change may lie in the impact of the Criminal Justice Act (1980) in Scotland. This changed police practice in respect of public drunkenness.

Drunken driving

The 1976 Report of the Government Committee on Drinking and Driving (the Blennerhasset Committee) gave an estimate of the total annual cost to this country of road accidents in which alcohol is involved. An estimated amount based on 1983 figures is an astonishing £178 million – a figure which includes damage to vehicles (and insurance claims), medical treatment of casualties, sickness benefits, police and court work, and so on. These are only the economic costs of drinking and driving. To audit the cost in terms of suffering and distress is more difficult. Detailed investigations of accidents by the Transport and Road Research Laboratory showed that in 1974 one in

Table 3   *Persons convicted of drunkenness offences in Britain, 1960–84*

| Year | England and Wales | | Scotland | |
	n	rate[a]	n	rate[a]
1960	68,109	19.3	8,520	22.0
1961	74,694	21.0	9,713	25.2
1962	83,992	23.3	9,996	25.8
1963	83,007	22.8	10,799	27.9
1964	76,842	21.0	10,778	27.9
1965	72,980	19.8	10,380	26.9
1966	70,499	19.0	10,620	27.6
1967	75,544	20.4	10,490	27.3
1968	79,070	21.2	10,937	28.6
1969	80,502	21.6	10,327	27.0
1970	82,374	22.0	10,594	27.6
1971	86,735	23.4	10,898	28.2
1972	90,198	24.0	11,664	30.5
1973	99,274	26.4	13,516	34.8
1974	103,203	27.4	14,683	37.5
1975	104,452	27.6	14,999	38.2
1976	108,698	28.6	14,156	35.8
1977	108,871	28.5	12,346	31.8
1978	106,814	27.8	12,643	32.4
1979	117,813	30.4	13,628	33.8
1980	122,259	31.4	13,795	29.8
1981	108,591	27.5	11,328	28.6
1982	107,326	27.1	9,730	23.7
1983	107,625	27.0	8.080	19.7
1984[1]	90,300	22.1	6,618	(16.5)

[a] Rate per 10,000 population aged 15 and over.

1. New cautioning procedures were introduced. This figure combines convictions for drunkenness with cautions.

Sources: Annual Home Office Reports, Scottish Home and Health Department annual crime statistics and the Brewers' Society UK Statistical Handbook, 1984.

three (about 900) drivers killed in road accidents had blood-alcohol levels above the statutory limit: between 10 p.m. and 4 a.m. on Monday to Friday the proportion of driver fatalities with levels over the legal limit rose to 51 per cent, and on Saturday nights to 71 per cent. In a survey of 2,000 road accidents, a drinking driver was involved in

25 per cent, and his condition deemed to be a major factor in 9 per cent. A more recent study by the same department indicated that 27 per cent of persons killed on the roads in England and Wales had blood-alcohol levels exceeding the United Kingdom legal limit of 80mg/100 millilitres. The corresponding Scottish proportion was markedly higher, at 53 per cent. Drinking significantly contributes to accidents of all degrees of severity, and perhaps particularly to the more serious accidents. Another obvious aspect of social cost is the tally of over 100,000 convictions for drunken driving in one year (1985), with costs to the police and to the courts, and many aspects of cost to the individual who almost invariably has his or her licence suspended.

As with alcohol and crime in general, the question which must immediately come to mind is whether we are sliding too easily towards an assumption of cause, when only statistical association is being demonstrated. This query will not only be raised, very properly, by the dispassionate critic who has a wary eye for this kind of logical error, but also by the drinkers who want to persuade themselves that personally their drinking only improves their driving. A mass of scientific evidence does, however, speak clearly of the causal nature of the demonstrated relationship.

The evidence comes partly from laboratory tests, which show the well-known impact of alcohol on reaction time. Such laboratory findings are far removed from the realities of the drive home on Saturday night, but it cannot be doubted that the physiological fact of impaired reaction time will have its practical effect when, after an evening in the pub, the driver suddenly has to make some fairly normal but split-second driving decision on which safety depends. A number of experiments on driving after drinking, conducted with volunteers, have shown the manner in which judgement and skill are actually affected.

But the most conclusive evidence comes from a survey conducted by the police department in Grand Rapids, Michigan, which obtained vital control information. Every person who had an accident had their blood-alcohol level assessed, and then control information was obtained by stopping motorists at the same accident points, and checking their blood-alcohol levels. This sort of data allows rejection of the argument that, at that time of night, a high percentage of all drivers will have been drinking. The Grand Rapids survey was able to give an estimate of the risk of being involved in an accident as a function of increased blood-alcohol level, compared to sober drivers in the control group. At 80mg per cent alcohol, the United Kingdom legal limit, the accident risk showed an increase approaching twice the sober risk level, by 150mg per cent the risk was ten times the normal, and by 200mg per cent the risk of accident was twenty times the normal level.

To argue the causal relationship between drinking and driving accidents is in no way to deny the multiple causes of most accidents, but only to highlight the fact that drinking frequently makes a major contribution to the mishap. Age and motoring experience are certainly also important, as are the driver's personality and alertness or fatigue. The road surface, lighting, and general driving conditions will bear on the likelihood of accident, as will the mechanical efficiency of the car, the behaviour of other drivers, and the behaviour of pedestrians. But the addition to a total situation of the driver's inebriety may often crucially tip the balance between safety and danger.

In 1967 the Road Traffic Act introduced the breathalyzer, and fixed the permitted statutory level of blood alcohol at 80mg per cent. Parliament rejected the notion of random breath testing. The act was preceded by an intensive publicity campaign. There is much evidence that the combination of new legislation, energetic enforcement, and public education produced immediate and dramatic effects. It has been calculated that about 5,000 lives were saved, and 200,000 casualties prevented in the first seven years of the act. Road casualties fell immediately by 11 per cent and deaths by 15 per cent. But over the ensuing years the effects of these measures were gradually eroded – the publicity was not sustained, the public seemed to forget the message, and various loopholes in the law hampered the task of enforcement. Above all individual drivers came to recognize that the chance of being stopped and breathalyzed was very small. In a recent survey 10 per cent of men admitted to driving regularly with their blood-alcohol over the legal limit. Table 4 shows recent trends in the number of people convicted of drunken driving in Britain. These numbers have risen dramatically since 1960 and this rise has far exceeded the growth of vehicle mileage. The rate of convictions for drunken driving is markedly higher in Scotland than in England and Wales. This disparity may be partly explained by differing police policies and road conditions. As shown by Table 4, Scottish convictions for drunken driving declined slightly between 1980 and 1983. In contrast, those south of the border have continued to rise. Approximately 95 per cent of those convicted of drunk driving are men.

No one can say how bad things would have been in the absence of the 1967 legislation, but certainly by 1974 the situation was again

Table 4   *Persons convicted of drunken driving in Britain, 1960–84*

year	England and Wales n	Scotland n	index of vehicle mileage[2]
1960	5,841	2,456	100
1961	6,502	2,866	109
1962	7,151	3,182	114
1963	7,474	3,536	121
1964	8,059	3,785	135
1965	8,857	4,213	145
1966	9,590	5,003	157
1967	10,038	5,363	164
1968[1]	18,374	5,597	172
1969	23,721	7,036	176
1970	26,273	8,413	186
1971	38,774	9,781	199
1972	47,098	10,158	209
1973	55,053	11,565	220
1974	56,153	12,201	215
1975	58,145	11,685	217
1976	49,999	9,621	228
1977	45,369	8,691	233
1978	49,695	10,450	243
1979	56,320	10,882	245
1980	66,394	12,513	261
1981	60,786	11,244	264
1982	63,832	10,429	276
1983	84,670	11,556	281
1984	101,000	12,213	——

1. The Road Safety Act came into effect on 9 October, 1967. This introduced the current 'breathalyzer' law.
2. Adapted from Road Research Laboratory's estimates of total vehicle mileage based on changes since 1960 base line.
Sources: Home Office, Scottish Health Department, Department of the Environment, Brewers' Society UK Statistical Handbook, 1984.

causing such official concern that a Government departmental committee was appointed. The Blennerhasset Committee reported in 1976, and made a variety of technical recommendations which, if introduced, would enable tighter enforcement. The burden of the committee's report was not that there should be more draconian punishment (or a lower statutory blood level), but that there should be movement towards a law that would allow a manifestly greater likelihood of apprehending and successfully prosecuting the offender. The notion of random breath testing is emotionally charged because of the fear of possible needless harassment, but the committee recommended more police discretion concerning the circumstances in which a driver may be asked to take a test. It is worth noting, too, that in some countries such as Finland random testing is well established and perfectly acceptable to the general public.

Technical advances in breath testing equipment mean that it is now possible for breath testing at the roadside followed by a breath test in the police station to be recommended as sufficient evidence for conviction, rather than incurring the delays and procedural uncertainties inherent in getting the police surgeon to conduct the additional statutory blood or urine test. Before May 1983 anyone who refused to give a sample of breath or whose test proved positive was normally required to give a blood or urine specimen. The procedure was changed as a result of the Transport Act (1981). Except in certain limited circumstances an evidential breath test, using electronic machines in police stations, replaced the blood or urine test. Between 6 May and 31 December 1983, 58,000 evidential breath tests were conducted, of which approximately 82 per cent were positive. This procedure is under review at present because of concern about the accuracy of the current apparatus for producing breath-test readings.

A recent review by the United States researcher, Professor H. Lawrence Ross, concluded that most traffic accidents in which alcohol plays a role do not, as popularly believed, involve moderate drinkers who simply happen to be 'unlucky'. Individuals who are convicted of drunken driving are not 'representative' of the general population: they are heavy drinkers. Ross noted: 'For example, in Sweden, the heaviest and presumably most tolerant users of alcohol accounted for 45 per cent of the alcohol-related crashes despite their comprising only 9 per cent of the general population.'

The realization that many drinking/driving offenders are regular heavy drinkers, particularly repeated offenders apprehended with very high blood-alcohol levels, has led to the institution of a procedure involving the Medical Adviser to the Driver and Vehicle

Licensing Department. 'High risk offenders', that is those convicted twice in a ten-year period with a blood-alcohol level of more than 200mg per cent, will need to demonstrate to the medical adviser that any underlying drink problem has been successfully dealt with before the licence is restored at the end of the second ban. Research is proceeding in a number of countries into whether intervention, such as education or training aimed at helping individuals limit their drinking, has a place in the sentencing of first offenders also.

PSYCHOLOGICAL DISABILITIES

Alcohol and mood

Alcohol may relieve unpleasant states of mind, and this will be discussed later in relation to the question of why people drink. But no drug taken to relieve deep-seated feelings of unease with life, self-doubt, or chronic tension will put those feelings right, except very transiently. Because alcohol is a drug to which tolerance develops, the likelihood is that alcohol will gradually be needed in larger and larger quantities, for the development of tolerance means that more of a drug is required to produce the same effects as before. Not only does drinking then begin to fail in its original purpose of relieving psychological distress and creating a happier mood, it begins to make matters worse. Heavy drinking itself begins to produce 'bad nerves' and the person concerned easily misinterprets this as a condition which requires further drink to put it right. Alcohol in large and continued quantities can itself produce a very depressing effect on mood, and the person becomes prey to all sorts of doubts, miseries, suspicions, and general gloom. He or she may also develop an acute fear of particular situations. This may be exacerbated by failing health, and the evident and undeniable accumulation of social problems which are legitimate causes for worry.

Heavy drinking thus easily leads to a state of mental distress which is not only misinterpreted by the subject, but which a doctor is apt to diagnose as 'depression' or 'anxiety' if the drinking history is missed. This is particularly true for female problem drinkers. Treatment with anti-depressants or tranquillizers will usually be ineffective, and can make matters worse. Minor tranquillizers are themselves potentially dependence-producing drugs. In addition they, like alcohol, are nervous system depressants, and are likely to compound the effects of alcohol and, more seriously, delay the formulation of the correct diagnosis.

This slow development of mental distress contributes to the appallingly high rates of suicide associated with alcohol dependence which is at least fifty times higher than in the general population. Much greater awareness of the role of alcohol in provoking suicide and attempted suicide is needed. A report from the Regional Poisoning Treatment Centre in Edinburgh showed that, in 1982, 40 per cent of all men admitted after taking an overdose were recorded as being excessive drinkers. The corresponding proportion among females was 16 per cent. Approximately a third of these excessive drinkers were alcohol dependent. The majority of alcohol dependent individuals who commit suicide are middle-aged and have been drinking for many years. It is noteworthy that many of these suicides occur within six weeks of experiencing an important loss, suggesting that this loss – of a friend or a job – was the last straw rendering life intolerable.

It should be realized that, as self-prescribed treatment for psychological problems, alcohol is a thoroughly dangerous medicine. Anyone who thinks he or she is drinking because of 'nerves' must also ask whether his or her 'nerves' are troubled because of drinking. To the medical profession it should be clear that 'bad nerves' or 'depression' should never be treated until enquiry has been made into the patient's drinking habits.

Alcohol and its influence on personality

As with its effect on mood, it has to be admitted that the personality problems which come from heavy drinking stem from an over-use of alcohol for purposes which are widely accepted. In a subtle way, one of the prime accepted uses of alcohol is to drink so that we will be rather different people. We will not only feel differently ourselves after a few drinks, but will act differently and be perceived differently by others. Drinking to harmonize interaction between people is likely to be at its maximum if both people are drinking rather than only one.

The hoped for cosmetic effect of drinking on personality is that it should make us jollier people, more confident, more extroverted, less guarded, more readily able to laugh, and generally better able to interact with other people. Our emotions are more readily available. We ourselves will feel more amusing, more powerful and important, and perhaps more sexually attractive.

The disadvantage may be that some of the effects of even moderate drinking on personality are not so attractive. Some people simply become bores. They are loquacious, and only want to talk about themselves. They may become boastful and silly. The supposed warmth of the interpersonal reactions can be a charade. All this may be irritating and distasteful to the member of the party who is more sober than the others, but it is generally more likely to be dreary than harmful. It is when such behaviour is regularly repeated, and someone who does not much like it has frequently to put up with it, that harm is done. This is what so often happens when one partner in a marriage is steadily or intermittently drinking to excess (the same issue has been discussed in a preceding section). A husband may be stupidly embarrassing at parties or in the pub. A wife is fed up with his boastfulness, silly stories, and pseudo-sexuality. He is perhaps attracted to the company of drinking friends who can enjoy the same superficialities and amount of alcohol. If she complains, there is a row. He claims to be hurt and sulks, and may then become abusive. The deterioration of behaviour towards friends, colleagues, employers, and neighbours gradually exhausts the heavy drinker's credit and destroys his or her reputation.

As the severity of a drinking problem and its chronicity advance, a person's previous personality may appear to be greatly altered for the worse, and hence the notion of 'personality deterioration'. When matters become as seemingly fixed as this, the more serious end of the spectrum has been reached. Friends will report that 'you simply can't believe anything he says'. This is not an inevitable consequence even of chronic, very heavy drinking, but in some degree it is not an uncommon picture. The drinker is then often labelled as suffering from 'severe personality disorder'. The development of this sort of situation is due to the toxic effects of alcohol. He repeatedly breaks his word because, when drinking is an imperative priority over all other considerations, he is in no position to keep his word. Brain substance may by then have been destroyed and intelligence, memory and particularly judgement seriously impaired.

Other mental disabilities

A frequent symptom of heavy drinking is a short-term amnesia or 'memory blackout'. In the morning the drinker cannot remember the events of the evening before, although during that evening he or she was fully conscious and behaving reasonably normally. This has sometimes been described as a certain sign of 'alcohol dependence', but is in fact a symptom which may have been experienced by 15 to 20 per cent of all individuals who drink:

A twenty-two-year-old representative of a whisky company came home from an evening drinking with friends. In the morning he had no recollection of coming home and seemed to have lost his car. He hired a taxi to take him looking for it and found it parked near a local discotheque. Friends said that he had been drinking but did not appear unduly drunk. They went on to enjoy further drinks and dancing later in the evening. He was persuaded to leave his car and take a taxi home. Friends claimed that he was active, coherent, and fully conscious throughout this episode but for him it was a total blank.

It is certainly a serious warning sign. With increasingly serious drinking, amnesias may begin to occur with greater frequency and even up to a few days of experience may be completely 'blacked out'. These happenings can be extremely frightening and perplexing for the person concerned. Recent research has been focusing on the brain mechanisms that are involved. It is evident that this defect in establishing lasting memory traces is most likely to occur when the blood-alcohol concentration is rising rapidly.

The mental complication of excessive drinking which is probably most widely known is *delirium tremens* (DTs) or 'the horrors'. The classical picture is easily recognized. The sufferer is obviously physically ill, very frightened, shaking, confused, and talking about hallucinations, visions, or voices. The picture is, however, not always so clear-cut, and can be mistaken for the delirium of pneumonia or the confusion of a post-operative state. DTs are likely to develop within a few days of alcohol withdrawal or a reduction in alcohol intake. *Withdrawal fits* may occur within about forty-eight hours of abstinence. Although full understanding of the underlying biochemical upsets in delirium tremens is still incomplete, this illness is to a large extent to be understood as an extreme manifestation of the withdrawal syndrome in someone who is highly dependent.

A severe form of alcohol-related mental illness which is not so well known is *alcoholic hallucinosis*: the sufferers go about their business and are not physically ill or confused, but they are hearing hallucinatory voices, often saying hurtful things. A third condition which must be put in the list of major mental disorders is *alcoholic dementia*, a disorder which will receive further note in the section on physical disorders (p. 98).

Drinking is often associated with the development of morbid jealousy in which the problem drinker comes to believe that their spouse is being unfaithful. The belief is often held with terrifying conviction and may lead to threats of violence and even murder. As has been mentioned in discussing alcohol-related crime, the person who is drinking heavily may act out otherwise controlled or subconscious sexual problems. *Gambling* and heavy drinking often go together, sometimes with each seeming to exacerbate the other, or at times one problem substituting for the other.

Heavy alcohol use and *misuse of other drugs* are frequently linked. The drinker complains of bad nerves and he or she may be prescribed tranquillizers and sleeping tablets which may be taken in addition to alcohol. This leads to the development of a serious additional habit. The nurse, doctor, or pharmacist who has a drinking problem is likely, for obvious reasons of availability, also to abuse drugs. The problem should largely be seen as that of the combined misuse of alcohol and prescribed or 'over the counter' drugs (sometimes with a disastrous combined overdose), but at times a troubled young person who takes illegal drugs may take them jointly with alcohol. Sometimes the story is of an adolescent who develops a drinking problem a few years after leaving school, starts to use glues, solvents, amphetamines, cannabis, or even heroin, and who then in his or her late twenties gives up illegal drugs only to encounter problems with drinking once again. Those who are concerned with the rehabilitation of young drug users are today well aware of the danger that an apparent recovery will be destroyed by the development of heavy drinking. The heavy drinker is frequently also a confirmed tobacco smoker. The problem of multiple drug abuse including alcohol is being encountered with increasing frequency.

PHYSICAL DISABILITIES

Alcohol can adversely affect physical health in several ways. People who drink too much may, for instance, neglect their diet, and consequently suffer from nutritional deficiencies. Alcohol can have a direct toxic effect on certain body tissues. The person who is intoxicated may suffer injury or harm others. The general neglect of health and the lowering of the body's resistance can lead to an increased susceptibility to intercurrent infections. Often more than one process operates at the same time. Indeed, excessive drinking can, in one way or another, damage nearly every organ and system of the body and lead to premature death. It is well known that alcohol-related deaths are substantially under-reported. However, recent changes in the reporting of such deaths should enable more accurate figures to be collected in future, as the mention of alcohol on a death certificate will no longer necessarily lead to a coroner's inquest.

While it has been traditionally assumed that alcohol-related physical damage only occurs following daily consumption of alcohol in excess of

80g per day (there are approximately 8g alcohol in a standard drink, see p. 43) for substantial periods of time, it has become increasingly evident that damage can occur in persons drinking regularly at a more moderate level. Equally it should be appreciated that alcohol-related physical damage does not inevitably develop even after years of abuse. Individual susceptibility to alcohol-related physical disease is probably determined by a number of genetic, constitutional and environmental factors, many of which are unknown. Several studies over the last forty years have suggested that women are probably more susceptible to the toxic effects of alcohol than men. Following a standard oral dose of alcohol, women achieve significantly higher blood-alcohol values than men because their total body water is significantly less. Tissue ethanol concentrations are correspondingly higher in women and it is reasonable to suppose that over a period of time this might result in earlier or more severe tissue damage. There is a suggestion that the presence of certain inborn biochemical factors might influence the rate at which alcohol-related damage develops in an otherwise susceptible individual. Ethnic origin would also seem to be an important factor in determining susceptibility to alcohol-related damage. Numerous other genetic markers of susceptibility to develop alcohol-related injury have been suggested but none has yet stood up to scientific scrutiny.

Liver damage

Almost everyone is aware that excessive drinking can sometimes result in the development of cirrhosis, a condition in which the liver becomes shrunken, hard and knobbly and may not function. This is an extremely serious and unpleasant condition, with a high expectation of death within a few years if the sufferer continues to drink. Both length of drinking history and level of consumption bear on the risk of liver damage – in effect, the concern has to be with 'lifetime' intake. Excess alcohol consumption can lead to the development of a wide spectrum of liver injury which is generally believed to progress from fatty liver to alcoholic hepatitis (inflammation) and then to cirrhosis (shrinking and scarring). Fatty change is the first and commonest liver abnormality seen, but although fat accumulation reflects a profound metabolic disturbance within the liver it is not necessarily harmful. Thus, although the development of fatty change is accompanied by enlargement of the liver and disturbance of liver function tests, symptoms are generally absent. The majority of individuals who are alcohol dependent will develop fatty change at some stage of their drinking career but less than one-third go on to develop more serious injury even after decades of alcohol abuse. In this susceptible group, alcoholic hepatitis, an acute inflammatory disorder, develops after five to fifteen years of drinking. This condition may produce little or no symptoms or else may be accompanied by a profound illness characterized by fever, abdominal pain, jaundice, bleeding into the gut, and coma. Alcoholic hepatitis may persist unchanged for some time but in a high percentage of patients the scar tissue laid down in the liver as part of the healing process leads to the development of cirrhosis. Patients with cirrhosis may also be largely symptom free, though abnormalities are present both on examination and in laboratory tests. On the other hand, these patients may be jaundiced and suffer from fluid retention, gastrointestinal bleeding, and episodic or persistent neuropsychiatric abnormalities. While the development of cirrhosis is usually associated with daily intakes of over 80g of alcohol in men and 50g in women, daily intakes of 40g (i.e. approximately four standard drinks per day) in men and 20g (approximately two standard drinks per day) in women have been linked with a significant increase in the risk of developing cirrhosis. Symptoms of liver disease may not appear for twenty years, but in some they may appear in as little as five. Up to 10 per cent of patients with alcoholic cirrhosis will develop liver cancer as a late complication of their disease.

A close association exists between per capita consumption of alcohol and cirrhotic deaths. Thus as alcohol consumption increases worldwide the death rates from cirrhosis climb in parallel. Indeed, in many countries the death rate from cirrhosis is rising while the overall death rate remains steady or falls.

At present there is no reliable way to predict which patients with alcohol-related fatty liver will eventually develop cirrhosis. Thus all patients with this condition should be advised to abstain from alcohol at least for an initial period of assessment. With abstinence the fatty liver will revert to normal within a few months and the outlook for the patient is excellent. Patients with mildly to moderately severe alcoholic hepatitis will also show significant improvement following abstinence from alcohol, though some will still eventually develop cirrhosis and die. Severe alcoholic hepatitis can be fatal but in those who survive the acute illness the long-term outlook is considerably improved by stopping drinking. Thus patients reducing their alcohol intake have an 80 per cent chance of surviving seven years whereas in those patients continuing to drink the seven year survival falls to 50 per cent. Similarly, the outlook for patients with alcoholic cirrhosis who stop drinking is significantly better than for their counterparts who continue to drink.

The important message for the patient with alcohol-related liver disease is that, if he or she goes on drinking, the liver condition will further deteriorate, with progressive invalidism and a much curtailed life expectancy. There are few circumstances in which abstinence can be so life saving. When a male patient stops drinking, the liver disease will often cease to progress. However, there is evidence that once liver disease has developed in a woman of child-bearing age, it may continue to progress even after drinking has been halted.

Drinking is by no means the only possible cause of cirrhosis, but over recent years alcoholic cirrhosis has in this country come to make a much larger contribution to the total cirrhosis death rate than was previously the case: in two studies conducted in Birmingham, the proportion of alcoholic cirrhosis rose from 33 per cent to 51 per cent of total cirrhosis cases, between 1959–64 and 1964–69. A study in South London showed alcoholic cirrhotics accounting for 65 per cent of the total. National figures of death from chronic liver disease and liver cirrhosis between 1970 and 1984 are shown in Table 5. The rate of mortality from these causes in Scotland is approximately twice that in England and Wales. The reasons for this surprising and long-standing difference are not clear.

Gastro-intestinal tract and nutrition

Alcohol increases the reflux of stomach contents into the oesophagus or gullet which may lead to inflammation and possible ulceration at the boundary between stomach and gullet. Violent retching or vomiting may produce a tear in the lining of this area and this can cause brisk and often profuse bleeding. The risk of developing cancer of the oesophagus is increased in those drinking 80g or more of alcohol daily and this risk is potentiated by the use of tobacco. Excessive drinking is also associated with an increased risk of cancer of the throat and mouth.

Alcohol may cause acute inflammation of the lining of the stomach, and this so-called acute gastritis is thought to account for the morning nausea and vomiting so commonly observed in drinkers and may itself be associated with gastric bleeding. Alcohol also causes chronic inflammation of the lining of the stomach in individuals abusing alcohol over long periods. The relationship between alcohol use and the development of ulcers in the stomach and duodenum is not clear. However, large amounts of alcohol will aggravate ulcers once present.

If large quantities of calories are taken as alcohol the diet generally becomes imbalanced, even if the quantity of food taken is considered adequate. Alcohol also directly interferes with the absorption and

Table 5   *Number and rate of deaths from chronic liver disease and liver cirrhosis in the United Kingdom, 1970–84*

year	England and Wales		Scotland	
	n	rate[1]	n	rate[1]
1970	1,392	2.8	239	4.6
1971	1,570	3.2	219	4.2
1972	1,662	3.4	258	5.0
1973	1,804	3.7	264	5.1
1974	1,754	3.6	328	6.3
1975	1,835	3.7	309	5.9
1976	1,890	3.8	319	6.1
1977	1,820	3.7	336	6.5
1978	1,926	3.9	382	7.4
1979	2,186	4.4	431	8.3
1980	2,218	4.5	406	7.8
1981	2,212	4.5	450	8.7
1982	2,152	4.4	422	8.2
1983	2,184	4.4	431	8.3
1984	2,280	4.6	423	8.2

1. Rate per 100,000 total population.
Sources: Annual Abstract of Statistics (London: HMSO). Common Services Agency, Scotland.

utilization of essential nutrients from food and as a result alcohol-dependent individuals are often malnourished. This may seriously affect their ability to cope with infection and illness and may limit their ability to repair the physical damage caused by alcohol.

Alcohol damages and may ultimately destroy the pancreas gland, an organ which produces secretions to aid digestion and the hormone insulin which is required for adequate control of blood sugar. When the function of this organ is impaired digestion is disturbed and diabetes may develop. The main symptom of pancreatic damage is pain which occurs in episodes, is usually severe and accompanied by vomiting and is often precipitated by a bout of drinking. Acute pancreatitis is predominantly a problem of heavy drinking young males. It has an immediate mortality of 9 per cent. Once damage is established the episodes of pain may continue despite abstinence from alcohol. Treatment of this condition is generally difficult and unsatisfactory.

Heart disease and hypertension

Alcohol can affect the function of heart muscle. Binge drinking may result in disturbances of heart rhythm in otherwise fit individuals who are not habitual drinkers. The rhythm disturbances may lead to palpitations or in the extreme to sudden death. Alcohol probably causes chronic disease of the heart muscle which initially may be reversible with abstinence from alcohol but which eventually progresses and leads to heart failure. More rarely heart disease may develop because of the heavy drinker's lack of vitamin B_1 (thiamine).

It has frequently been noted that there appears to be a lower incidence of cardiovascular deaths in patients who drink a little alcohol compared with those who either take none or larger quantities. This may, of course, reflect the fact that heavy drinkers do not live long enough to develop serious cardiovascular disease and at the other extreme abstainers may have chosen this way of life because of pre-existing ailments that contribute to early death.

In 1974, the Department of Health, Education and Welfare's report to the United States Congress suggested that moderate drinkers were likely to suffer fewer heart attacks than those who had stopped drinking, drank too much, or drank not at all. They based their assertion in part on a study at the Kaiser-Permanente Medical Centre in Oakland, California which consulted the histories of 120,000 patients and found that moderate alcohol users were 30 per cent less likely to suffer heart attacks than non-drinkers. A similar study in Honolulu of 7,705 Japanese men reached similar conclusions. These men had been divided into three groups and the incidence of heart attacks per 1,000 calculated. Ex-drinkers showed a rate of 56:1,000, life-long teetotallers a rate of 44:1,000 and current drinkers a rate of 30:1,000.

Since these early studies which suggested that alcohol in moderate amounts (approximately two standard units daily) might possibly protect against coronary heart disease, many more studies have been published which support the suggestion, refute the suggestion, or else were too inconclusive to allow comment on the suggestion.

If alcohol in moderate doses does indeed convey a protective effect against the risk of developing coronary heart disease, the mechanism by which this effect is brought about needs exploring. At present the question as to whether alcohol in moderate amounts protects the heart in some way is unproven and must remain open for debate. What has become clear, however, from many studies is that individuals regularly consuming alcohol show no improvement in general health since they die more often of strokes, cancer, accidents, and violence. It has in fact been suggested that any apparent good effect on the heart might be explained on the basis of the competing risk phenomenon. That is, that individuals drinking alcohol regularly would develop coronary artery disease if they did not die prematurely from other causes. However persuasive the argument that alcohol taken in moderation produces true or perceived benefit, the fact remains that taken in excess it produces incalculable harm.

There is a close relationship between blood pressure readings and reported alcohol intake. Thus less than 10 per cent of abstainers or light drinkers show elevated blood pressure compared with more than 20 per cent of those consuming 120g alcohol per day. Indeed excess alcohol intake is now regarded as the commonest identifiable, causal factor of elevated blood pressure in young men. Excess alcohol intake has been implicated in the development of strokes, especially in young people. In fact strokes are three times commoner in heavy drinkers. They appear to be particularly closely associated with occasions of excessive drinking, possibly because of the effects of alcohol on blood clotting or on blood pressure. A link has also been identified between excessive drinking and bleeding into the spaces around and within the brain (i.e. subarachnoid haemorrhage).

Brain and nervous system

The behavioural results of alcohol intoxication do not require detailing. Suffice to say that with increasing intoxication, speech becomes slurred, co-ordination, reasoning and memory become increasingly impaired, and drowsiness advances. Death may result from respiratory depression or at an earlier stage of intoxication from inhalation of vomit. The blood-alcohol levels necessary to produce intoxication depend on the degree of tolerance acquired by previous regular consumption of alcohol. Thus in non-habitual drinkers, blood-alcohol concentrations of 150–200mg per cent generally give rise to obvious intoxication, while in regular very heavy drinkers concentrations of 300mg per cent may be present without evidence of intoxication.

Prolonged alcohol abuse is also associated with some specific forms of brain damage. Best known are Wernicke's encephalopathy and Korsakoff's psychosis, both of which occur as a result of deficiency of the vitamin thiamine. Sufferers from Wernicke's encephalopathy manifest mental and behavioural changes, paralysis of eye movement, and unsteadiness. Korsakoff's psychosis is characterized by profound impairment of memory for recent events. In practice, these two conditions overlap to a large degree. If recognized early the response to treatment with the vitamin thiamine is good. Sadly the diagnosis is often missed in life and only discovered at postmortem.

More generalized brain damage also occurs among patients clinically defined as alcohol dependent. There can be no doubt that excessive drinkers with apparently intact general intelligence show specific abnormalities when their mental processes are tested and show evidence of loss of brain tissue on brain scan (a radiographic technique that displays the shape of the brain). However, the appearance of the brain scan improves following abstinence and some improvement occurs in brain functioning. The changes in mental functioning detected by psychological testing can be quite subtle, involving difficulties in abstract reasoning, learning new skills, and coping with complex visuospatial problems. For example, a worker for a furniture firm found that he lost the ability to pack and store furniture in a van because he could no longer envisage its positioning within the available space. These deficits often improve after three or four weeks abstinence and continuing improvement is sometimes evident for a year or more after cessation of drinking. The treatment implications of these observations will be considered in a later chapter.

Individuals who are alcohol dependent are also prone to develop abnormalities in the nerves supplying the limbs, which result in difficulties in movement and impairment of sensation. This peripheral neuropathy, as it is called, may or may not be related to vitamin deficiencies. Although a good deal of recovery is possible following abstinence from alcohol, many patients are left with intractable pain or unpleasant sensations in their limbs, mainly the legs. Acute muscle weakness and pain – myopathy – is also a well-recognized but unusual complication of a prolonged heavy drinking bout. Chronic damage to muscles may occur in individuals misusing alcohol over long periods and manifests as muscle weakness and wasting.

Accidents and trauma

The relationship between drinking and road accidents has been discussed earlier in this chapter, and it is clear that there is an increased accident risk at levels of drinking well within the social-drinking range. There is not nearly so much hard information on the relationship between drinking levels and accidents in the home or factory. In one study of 300 consecutive fatalities from unintentional injuries, however, 30 per cent of those dying were known to be heavy drinkers. A report from the Western Infirmary in Glasgow has shown that almost 50 per cent of the admissions for head injuries are the result of assaults or falls while under the influence of alcohol and, at that hospital, admissions for such injuries are currently running at about 1,000 a year. In a later and more intensive study also conducted at the Western Infirmary, 62 per cent of all males admitted with head injury were found to have alcohol in their blood, but it was not so much the presence but the level of alcohol which was astonishing: the average blood-alcohol level of those who had been drinking was 193mg per cent or two-and-a-half times the legal driving limit.

The Royal Life Saving Society has, for several years, noted in its annual reports that alcohol is the commonest single factor in death by drowning. In 1984, drinking was implicated in 19 per cent of such deaths. In addition a report produced by the Department of Trade and Industry in 1977 noted that alcohol consumption was a factor in 43 per cent of deaths from falls and in 39 per cent of deaths from fires. The Consumer Safety Unit at the Trade and Industry Department also reported that 30 per cent of accidental deaths in the 51–64 age group involved alcohol.

Effects on sexual function

It is well known that intoxication may impair sexual performance. The association between chronic alcohol abuse and disorders of sexual function in men has been known for centuries. These men lose sexual drive and potency, their testes and penis may shrivel, and they produce very little semen containing few sperms. The incidence of these changes varies: 40–90 per cent report loss of libido while 10–75 per cent show reduction in the size of their testes. Men who maintain a very high level of alcohol consumption may also become feminized; many lose body hair and up to 60 per cent develop an increase in breast tissue.

Female problem drinkers often have sexual difficulties and experience loss of menstruation, menstrual cycle irregularities, or heavy menstrual loss. In addition, up to 75 per cent lose breast tissue; sex organs may reduce in size and the vagina may become dry.

Very little is known about the reversibility of the effects of alcohol on sexual function; the only information available relates to male alcoholics. Impotence will improve in 25–50 per cent of male drinkers who subsequently abstain from alcohol. However, alcoholic men showing severe reduction in the size of their testes are unlikely to regain adequate sexual functioning despite prolonged abstinence from alcohol.

Recently, it has been shown that the ingestion of even moderate amounts of alcohol may also cause male infertility. Thus of 90 men attending a male infertility clinic 40 per cent were thought to have low sperm counts as a result of drinking 30–50g alcohol per day (2–3 pints of beer). Prompt return of the sperm counts to normal was observed in approximately half the men who subsequently abstained. No information is available on the effects of moderate alcohol consumption on female fertility.

Effects on the fetus

Concern about the effects of maternal drinking during pregnancy has been evident since ancient times. In Sparta and Carthage couples were prohibited from drinking on their wedding night in order to protect any children conceived at this time. In 1726 the College of Physicians reported to Parliament that parental drinking was responsible for 'weak, feeble and distempered children'. During the past twenty years there has been a resurgence of concern about this topic. A considerable body of animal research shows that maternal use of alcohol (like many other drugs) may harm fetal development. In addition, it has been reported that women who drink heavily during pregnancy also risk harming their offspring. Researchers in Seattle coined the term 'fetal alcohol syndrome' to describe babies who had been harmed by their mothers' drinking during pregnancy. Such children had a characteristic cluster of facial features as well as stunted growth, physical disabilities, and intellectual impairment. It has been suggested that although the fully-fledged syndrome is rather rare, lesser forms of harm may be more commonplace and might be associated with lower levels of alcohol consumption. In 1981, the United States Surgeon General issued a forceful warning about the dangers of drinking during pregnancy. Since then this issue has been hotly debated. Several follow-up studies of pregnant women have now been completed. Many of these show that while maternal drinking during pregnancy is *associated* with birth abnormalities, so too are other factors, some of which appear to be far more important than alcohol. These include maternal age, social class, tobacco, illegal drug and medicine use, obstetric history, and diet. Most pregnant women do not drink heavily and the majority of available evidence does not suggest that 'moderate' consumption, for example, one or two standard drinks once or twice a week, has any harmful effects upon fetal development.

Women who drink heavily or who are alcohol dependent may well increase their risks of producing damaged offspring. Even so the fetal alcohol syndrome appears to be rare in the United Kingdom and is probably the result of a combination of many factors of which alcohol is only one. The best advice for women who are either pregnant or who are contemplating pregnancy is to minimize their use of both alcohol and other psychoactive drugs, never to become intoxicated, and never to consume more than one or two standard units of alcohol (see p. 43) more than once or twice a week.

Prevalence of drinking problems in general hospitals

In view of the array of harmful physical consequences associated with excess consumption, it is hardly surprising that as many as one-quarter of the men and a sizeable minority of women in general medical and surgical wards will be found to have alcohol-related problems. A recent study of casualty attenders found that 32 per cent had excessive levels of alcohol in their blood. This prevalence underlines the importance of doctors enquiring about alcohol consumption among hospital patients.

Mortality studies

The question of whether abstinence is associated with longevity has been much debated for well over a century. A recent review has concluded that abstainers appear not to live quite as long as those who drink very moderately. However, even the heavier types of 'acceptable social drinking' carry some probability of a shortened life. There is certainly a high mortality rate among heavy drinkers clinically identified as alcohol dependent. A recent British publication reported a death-certificate search on a group of 935 patients who had been admitted to mental hospitals with a diagnosis of alcohol dependence, and who were followed up after ten to fifteen years. The actual death rate exceeded that which would have been expected in a general population group of the same age by a factor of 2.7 for men and 3.1 for women. Among subjects aged below forty years, this factor was 9.2. Considering different causes of death separately, the factor was 3.1 for tuberculosis, 1.7 for cancers, 22.7 for cirrhosis of the liver, and 24.9 for suicide. For accidents, poisoning and violence combined the factor was 15.8.

Economic costs of alcohol-related problems

The adverse effects of alcohol misuse impose a significant economic burden on society. Reference has already been made to the cost of drunken driving. It would never be possible to place any reliable economic value on adverse effects such as broken homes and disturbed children. Moreover, only limited information exists about the economic cost of alcohol misuse even in relation to important spheres such as industrial productivity, absenteeism, and accidents. A recent review conservatively concluded that the annual cost of alcohol misuse in England and Wales (at 1983 prices) was in excess of £1,500 million. The costs for Northern Ireland and Scotland are proportionately greater since levels of alcohol misuse appear to be rather higher in these parts of the United Kingdom. A summary of the toll of alcohol misuse in England and Wales is presented in Table 6.

Table 6   *Total costs of alcohol misuse in England and Wales, 1983*

category	cost in £ millions
social cost to industry	1396.8
social cost to National Health Service	95.9
expenditure on national alcohol agencies and research	1.0
traffic accidents	89.2
criminal activities	32.2

Source: McDonnel and Maynard, 1985: 33.

SOME IMPLICATIONS

We started this chapter by saying that its concern would be to display and examine the wide array of minor or major problems, mishaps or damage in which drinking can be a causal or contributing factor. It was no part of that intention to over-dramatize; and it is again worth emphasizing that the majority of people who drink moderately will rarely come to any resultant harm. But on the basis of all the material accumulated in this chapter it must now be equally obvious that alcohol misuse can result in disabilities of astonishing diversity, that these disabilities range from the trivial to the crippling or fatal, and that frequently when figures can be produced the contribution that alcohol is making to varieties of incapacity is of major and surprising significance. The picture must not be luridly exaggerated, but at present the danger of imbalance largely lies in the other direction – most people in this country will today have only the haziest idea as to the true costs of excessive drinking in misery, illness, and death. Nor will they have any awareness of the financial costs involved. Fragments of information on this or that aspect of the problem have found their way into public consciousness, but what is so lacking is an awareness of the startling pattern that emerges when all these separate bits of information are put together.

The total picture which is portrayed here must be made more common public property. We have presented evidence in Chapter 3 of this Report to support the optimistic belief that awareness has grown over the past two or three decades, but the level of awareness in general still falls far short of that which the facts properly demand. And the nature of those facts directly supports the argument that the need is for the widest possible community awareness, for it is every aspect of the community's life that is affected by excessive drinking. The scenes of our concern must embrace houses, streets, schools, offices and factories, courts and prisons, as well as consulting rooms, casualty departments, and hospital wards. It must include the families and children, neighbours, workmates, and the other road users, who are inevitably and repeatedly going to be involved – for it is almost inconceivable that a drinking problem would affect only one actor, or only one actor and a single therapist or other 'helper'.

For the helping professions and the design of services the evidence implies the importance of being able to respond to an extraordinarily wide variety of problems, and which should often be able to deal with the alcohol issue within a wider and unspecialized context of causes and disorders. It must be obvious that a specialized treatment service which sits back and waits for the problem to present itself as alcohol dependence will only be able to make a tiny contribution to what is really needed.

A further implication relates to prevention. What has to be prevented is clearly not one single type of process, one disease entity of 'alcoholism', or anything of unitary causation, but a mass of problems of varied origin in the genesis of which alcohol plays a greater or lesser contributing part. Insights that come from this type of review must lead to broad but well directed and multiple preventative strategies.

The final implication to be drawn must be that there are still manifest gaps in the evidence. So far, there has been little in the way of purposive and comprehensive monitoring of the social, health, and economic costs of excessive drinking. Small pieces of evidence from that city or this hospital, supported perhaps by mortality statistics or crime statistics, allow some sort of patchwork to be put together. But the information is often incomplete, and it is most often available only because of the chance zeal of some particular investigator. We should demand to know more often and more completely.

7

Social causes of harmful drinking

The nature of alcohol dependence was discussed in Chapter 5 and the wide range of social problems and medical disorders which can result from excessive drinking was described in Chapter 6. The question which now has to be tackled is why people drink alcohol, why they drink as much, or as little, as they do, and what relationship there is between the amount they drink and the risk that their drinking will have harmful consequences. These are complicated as well as important issues. It may be helpful, therefore, to discuss the many factors influencing consumption patterns and their associated ill effects under the two broad headings of environmental (or social) and personal (or individual) factors, despite the fact that the two are in constant interaction with one another.

THE SOCIAL AND OTHER ENVIRONMENTAL FACTORS INFLUENCING CONSUMPTION

Alcoholic drinks are available, or could readily be so, in almost all contemporary societies, and have been available in most of them for hundreds or even thousands of years. Despite this ubiquity the quantity of alcohol consumed varies greatly from one country to another, from one social group to another, and from one generation to another. Some of the more striking global and historical differences have already been referred to in Chapter 2. These differences are important for two reasons. First because, just as the more an individual drinks the more likely he or she is to suffer ill effects of one sort or another, so the more a community or nation drinks the greater are the adverse effects suffered by that community or nation. Secondly, because the existence of major differences in the drinking patterns and levels of consumption of different countries and social groups, and changes in these from one generation to the next, make it clear that there is nothing immutable about our own contemporary drinking patterns and consumption levels. In ten or twenty years time we might be drinking more than we do now, or we might be drinking less. If in future we drink more than at present the medical and social ill effects we suffer will almost certainly be even greater than they are now, and if we drink less these ill effects will almost certainly be diminished.

The relationship between national consumption levels and the ill effects of alcohol

The drinking habits of the members of a community or of the inhabitants of a country are often extremely varied. Some people never drink alcohol at all, others only do so on rare occasions like Christmas or the New Year, or at weddings. Others drink some alcohol most weeks. Others drink a great deal nearly every day. And most people's consumption varies from day to day and month to month. However, if a representative sample of the adult members of a population are interviewed and questioned in detail about their drinking habits it is almost invariably found that most people drink relatively moderately but that a minority drinks very large quantities. In fact the distribution of consumption in a population nearly always takes the form shown in Figure 2. The consumption curve is continuous, unimodal, and skewed towards the right hand (high consumption) end. It is important to note that there is no discontinuity between the moderate drinkers in the centre and the excessive drinkers at the right hand side, a fundamental fact we will return to subsequently.

Information about people's drinking habits can, of course, only be obtained by personal enquiry. There is no convenient blood test providing a measure of how much someone is accustomed to drinking, or has drunk in the last week or two. Measuring the amount of alcohol in blood, or in expired air with a breathalyzer, provides a fairly accurate measure of how much has been drunk within the last few hours, but only over this brief time period. However, while moderately raised blood-alcohol concentrations may be found in occasional as well as habitual drinkers, detection of higher values are more suggestive of habitual drinking. Thus, a blood-alcohol level above 100mg per cent without intoxication or above 300mg per cent at any time can be regarded as highly suggestive of chronic alcohol abuse.

Usually in surveys people are asked what they drink in a typical week or a typical month, or what they have actually drunk in the last seven days. Sometimes they cannot remember and heavier drinkers will often

Figure 2 *Typical distribution of different levels of alcohol consumption in a population*

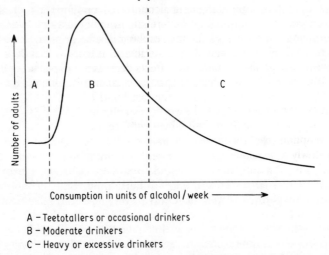

A – Teetotallers or occasional drinkers
B – Moderate drinkers
C – Heavy or excessive drinkers

not admit how much they really drink. Indeed, it is well known that estimates of total population consumption obtained in this way from surveys rarely account for much more than half of the alcohol which sales information or Customs and Excise returns indicate has actually been consumed. Nevertheless, surveys and questionnaire responses are widely used for estimating who drinks how much and on what occasions and the results are usually fairly reliable and consistent from one survey to another. Response rates are probably a key factor in reliability and consistency from one survey to another.

In Britain and most other industrial countries Customs and Excise returns, although they do not provide any information about individual consumption, do provide a fairly accurate measure of the total quantity of alcohol consumed in the country each year. Home brewing and duty free imports by returning travellers are missed, of course, but in Britain at present they only account for a very small proportion of total consumption. Consequently, consumption per head of population (the total quantity of alcohol consumed divided by the total population or, more usefully, by the total adult population) is a fairly accurate and readily available measure of average consumption levels. In the United Kingdom in 1984, for example, consumption per person aged 15 and over was 9.2 litres (about 16.1 pints) of absolute alcohol. In other words, the average adult drank about two gallons of pure alcohol in the course of the year (equivalent to 439 pints of beer or 31 bottles of spirits).

One of the cardinal facts about alcohol from a public health point of view is that there is a close relationship between per capita consumption and the scale of the resulting ill effects. If consumption per head rises all the readily measurable ill effects also rise, and if consumption per head falls the ill effects decrease. This relationship is well illustrated by the changes that have taken place in the United Kingdom's consumption during the last hundred years. These have been described earlier but are worth restating in this context.

In the second half of the nineteenth century United Kingdom consumption rose to extremely high levels, but after 1900 it started to fall, slowly at first and then very rapidly during the First World War, largely as a result of the controls imposed by Lloyd George's government. There was a further fall during the great depression of the 1930s. Table 7 shows the effect of these changes in per capita consumption on a rough index of alcohol-related mortality, derived from the number of death certificates each year reporting the cause of death as chronic alcoholism, delirium tremens, or cirrhosis of the liver. While consumption was still rising, between 1885 and 1900, mortality rose. But as soon as consumption started to fall alcohol-related

Table 7   *United Kingdom alcohol consumption per head of population and alcohol-related mortality for quinquennial periods 1885–1930*

quinquennium	average annual per capita consumption (in litres of absolute alcohol)	average annual deaths per million living certified as due to chronic alcoholism, DTs or cirrhosis
1885–89	9.9	154
1890–94	10.4	168
1895–99	10.9	182
1900–4	10.6	193
1905–9	9.3	156
1910–14	8.8	131
1915–19	6.0	81
1920–24	6.0	59
1925–29	5.2	55
1930–34	4.2	42

mortality did likewise, slowly at first but increasing rapidly as consumption fell more and more. Part of this fall in mortality was probably due to slow improvements in medical care and the index is in any case rather crude, for alcohol contributes directly or indirectly to many deaths without ever figuring on the death certificate. None the less, the relationship between changes in consumption and changes in mortality is close and impressive.

After the Second World War United Kingdom consumption started to rise again, slowly at first but more rapidly in the 1960s and 1970s. Our consumption almost doubled between 1950 and the mid-1970s, from 5.2 litres of absolute alcohol per person aged 15 or over in 1950 to 9.3 litres in 1976. Over this time period there was a steep rise in the incidence of three well-known and relatively well-documented consequences of excessive drinking – convictions for public drunkenness, deaths from cirrhosis of the liver, and mental hospital admissions with a primary diagnosis of alcoholism. Hospital admissions for alcoholism rose very steeply indeed, partly because treatment facilities were being increased in an attempt to meet the newly acknowledged and increasing need.

Between 1979 and 1982 United Kingdom consumption fell somewhat, mainly because of the effect of the recession on consumer spending together with an increase in the excise duty on beer and spirits in the 1981 budget. Although the fall in per capita consumption over this three-year period was only 11 per cent it was sufficient to produce an almost immediate reduction in adverse effects. As Table 8 shows, between 1980 and 1982 first admissions for alcohol dependence fell by 19 per cent, drunkenness convictions fell by 16 per cent, drinking and driving convictions fell by 7 per cent, and cirrhosis mortality fell by 4 per cent. Similar changes have been reported in other countries. Indeed, it is very nearly true to say that there is no well-documented instance in the alcohol literature over the last hundred years of a major change taking place in a country's per capita consumption without corresponding changes taking place in the incidence of the adverse effects of excessive drinking.

There is, of course, no law of nature decreeing that all these adverse effects must increase if consumption per head of population increases, and vice versa. It is perfectly possible to envisage a situation in which cirrhosis mortality might actually fall, despite an increase in consumption, because of improvements in the medical treatment of cirrhosis, or a situation in which drunkenness convictions rose despite a fall in consumption because of a change in the policy of the courts or the police. In practice the relationship between consumption per head and

Table 8   *United Kingdom alcohol consumption per head of population and convictions for public drunkenness, drinking and driving convictions, cirrhosis mortality and hospital admissions for alcohol dependence, 1970–84*

year	UK alcohol consumption per head in litres of pure alcohol	UK drunkenness convictions per 10,000 pop.	drinking and driving con- victions in Britain per 10,000 pop.	cirrhosis deaths in England and Wales per 100,000 pop.	English hospital first admissions for alcohol dependence per 100,000 pop.
1970	7.03	22.3	8.4	3.71	5.17
1971	7.37	23.4	11.7	4.19	5.70
1972	7.79	24.1	13.8	4.41	6.19
1973	8.61	26.6	16.0	4.77	7.34
1974	8.85	27.7	16.3	4.63	8.11
1975	8.82	27.9	16.6	4.82	8.40
1976	9.28	28.6	14.1	4.94	8.68
1977	8.81	28.2	12.7	4.73	9.17
1978	9.50	27.5	14.1	4.97	9.13
1979	9.79	29.9	15.6	5.60	9.74
1980	9.33	30.9	18.2	5.64	10.96
1981	8.89	27.1	16.5	5.59	10.55
1982	8.67	26.1	17.0	5.42	8.91
1983	8.83	25.7[1]	22.3[2]	5.47	8.63
1984	9.21	22.1[1]	22.8	5.67	9.46

Note: All figures refer to the population aged fifteen or over. The per capita consumption figures are slightly different from those in Table 1 because of slightly different assumptions about the average alcohol content of beers and wines, and because they refer to calendar rather than fiscal years.

1. These figures are for England and Wales only.
2. The 1981 Road Transport Act introduced evidential breath-testing machines in May 1983.

cirrhosis mortality is remarkably close, so close that a country's cirrhosis mortality has sometimes been used as a means of estimating the quantity of alcohol its citizens consumed in situations in which no official figures were available. The relationship between consumption and other ill effects is looser, for a variety of reasons. Drinking and driving convictions are obviously influenced by the number of cars on the road as well as by the behaviour of drivers and policemen, and hospital admissions are influenced by bed availability and hospital policies as well as by the willingness of alcoholics to come forward for treatment. So minor increases or decreases in consumption sometimes take place without any change, or even a paradoxical change, in drunkenness convictions or hospital admissions. And for many of the most important harmful effects of drinking, like those on family life or on industrial accident rates, there simply are no figures available to indicate the direction of change. Despite these various caveats, however, the fact remains that in practice most of the easily measurable ill effects of excessive drinking, both medical and social, rise and fall predictably with changes in the quantity of alcohol consumed each year by the average citizen. Or to put it the other way about, consumption per head is the crucial variable determining the scale of the whole range of ill effects resulting from excessive drinking.

Why should this be? The explanation is that the population is not composed of two separate groups, a large one of 'normal social drinkers' whose drinking habits are harmless and a much smaller one of 'alcoholics' who are responsible for all the trouble. It is composed, as Figure 1 shows, of a broad spectrum of men and women drinking very varied amounts. The more an individual habitually drinks, the greater the likelihood of developing cirrhosis, of being involved in accidents, of losing his job, of becoming physically dependent on alcohol, and so on. But a substantial proportion of the ill effects are generated by quite moderate drinkers. A young man may drown swimming in the sea, or crash his car, simply because he has unwisely drunk four pints of beer for lunch, and a middle-aged woman may suffer burns when she falls deeply asleep after three whiskies and neglects her lighted cigarette. The chances of their doing so are small in comparison with those who drink two or three times as much. But because relatively moderate drinkers are so much more numerous than those who drink a bottle of gin or ten pints of beer a day, between them they still account for a high proportion of the ill effects.

It is also important to appreciate that people's drinking habits are constantly changing. Both men and women usually drink less after marriage than they did before. Job changes, particularly into or out of high risk occupations like the hotel and restaurant trades, the merchant navy, and the alcohol industry itself, are often associated with major changes in consumption. The breakdown of a marriage, the death of a relative, or a change in financial circumstances may also have major effects. For all these reasons it is quite wrong and very misleading to imagine that almost all the harm is caused by a small proportion of the population who are 'alcoholics', and different from the rest of us. Changes in total or per capita consumption, in either direction, are usually generated by changes throughout the spectrum of drinkers. When consumption per head was rising in the 1960s and 1970s it was doing so because everyone was tending to drink rather more. Occasional drinkers were tending to have a drink more frequently, those who had previously had one or two drinks once or twice a week were now having two or three drinks two or three times a week, and so on. Everyone tended to move slightly to the right on the spectrum illustrated in Figure 2. As a result the risk that their drinking might have harmful consequences, for themselves or other people, small though it might have been, increased somewhat. And, of course, some of those who were already rather heavy drinkers increased their intake a little more and so started to become dependent, or to develop the silent insidiously progressive internal changes that lead to cirrhosis or pancreatitis.

A very similar set of changes occurs in reverse when per capita consumption is falling. Everyone tends to drink a little less, they shift to the left on the spectrum and their personal risk is reduced. In particular those who were in, or about to enter, the danger zone for developing dependence or dying from cirrhosis move out of it, even though their consumption may remain relatively high. There may well be a small core of heavily dependent drinkers whose consumption does not fall at all, and who therefore remain at very high risk of further damage of various kinds. But because they are relatively few in number their behaviour does not prevent the incidence of most ill effects from falling in the population as a whole.

There are two main reasons why changes in total population consumption, both upwards and downwards, tend to involve most people who drink at all – occasional, moderate, and heavy drinkers. The first is that the major cause of the change, whether it be a change in legislation or in the excise duty on alcoholic beverages or in the country's overall economic prosperity, usually affects everyone. The second is what is sometimes called the 'snowball effect'. Most drinking is primarily social. If a man's friends or colleagues start to drink more they are more likely to offer him a drink if he calls on them at home, more likely to serve wine with a meal when entertaining, more likely to suggest meeting in a pub, and more likely to want to stay for a second drink when they do so. These changes in their behaviour lead him to drink more, and may also make him feel under an obligation to return their hospitality. So his habits start to change and then perhaps have further effects on theirs.

The implications of this close relationship between a community's or a country's per capita consumption and the scale of the ensuing ill effects, human, social, and economic, are very different from, and much less comfortable than, those of our previous assumptions. For the last fifty years it has been received wisdom that alcoholism is a disease, and that those unfortunates who become 'alcoholics' are in some way different from the rest of us. Whether for psychological or for biochemical reasons they were incapable of drinking moderately or sensibly and if they were unwise enough to continue drinking after their problems had been detected they got into all kinds of trouble. Despite the fact that hereditary influences undoubtedly play some part in the development of drinking problems, there never was much evidence to substantiate this view of the matter. It owed much of its popularity and wide currency to the fact that it was in almost everyone's interests to believe that alcoholics were different from other people. It left most people free to assume that their own drinking was as harmless as it was enjoyable. It left the alcohol industry free to advertise and sell its wares, and increase its sales, without any suggestion that this might be harmful. It even provided alcoholics with the comforting thought that they were ill, rather than merely weak-willed, and that it was someone else's responsibility – the medical profession's – to cure them.

Unfortunately, as we have seen, the facts do not fit these convenient assumptions. The reality is that almost anyone's drinking may get out of hand, with potentially dire consequences for themselves or other people, and whether it does so or not depends far more on how much they drink over how long a period than on their personality or their biochemistry. What is more, everyone's drinking contributes to the total quantity of alcohol consumed, and so there is an important sense in which anyone who drinks at all heavily, or increases his or her consumption from one year to the next, is contributing to the burden of harm borne by the community as a whole, whether or not they themselves suffer any immediate ill effects. Where drinking is concerned, as with other things, no one 'is an island entire of itself'. Another important implication is that all alcoholic drinks are equally dangerous, because it is the alcohol content which matters, rather than the unique qualities of that particular drink. The widespread belief that cider and beer are comparatively safe and that only spirits drinkers become alcoholics or develop cirrhosis is quite without foundation. In fact the majority of so-called alcoholics are beer drinkers, simply because beer is the predominant drink of British men, though less exclusively so than a generation ago. The only sense in which spirits are genuinely more dangerous than beer or wine is that, because their alcohol content is higher, it is easier to get drunk very quickly.

The social determinants of per capita consumption

As the total quantity of alcohol consumed per head of population per year is the crucial determinant of the level of harm, medical and social, resulting from excessive drinking it is obviously important to understand the many factors liable to influence consumption levels. They are conveniently divided into those which influence the demand for alcoholic beverages and those which influence their availability (see Table 9). Demand is primarily determined by cultural and religious traditions which differ considerably from place to place, and are largely responsible for the striking differences in consumption patterns to be found in different parts of the world. Arabs drink much less than Europeans mainly because the Muslim faith forbids any use of alcohol, so any drinking that does occur usually has to be in private. The French drink far more wine than the British because their climate allows them to grow vines which are a staple crop. They therefore regard wine as a food, and the natural accompaniment to meals, whereas for us it is, or used to be, the symbol of a special occasion. The French drink throughout the day, we drink mainly in the evenings and at weekends.

Table 9   *The major determinants of the quantity of alcohol consumed by a population*

---

1. *factors influencing demand*
   cultural and religious traditions
   consumer purchasing power
   advertising?
   health education?
2. *factors influencing availability*
   size of harvests and agricultural controls
   volume of beverage produced and/or imported and controls on these
   number and opening hours of retail outlets and controls on these
       (licensed premises and licensing hours)
   controls on purchasers (the age limit)
   price of alcoholic beverages and special taxes on these

The way in which such cultural differences develop is intriguing and poorly understood, for they are the result of a complex interplay between religious and economic forces, climate, and the lingering influence of earlier rulers, invaders, and merchants. For most practical purposes they are best regarded as the framework within which other factors operate, for they are, almost by definition, slow to change. Nor are they easily manipulated, as health educators have discovered. Availability, on the other hand, may change, as a result of war or the failure of a harvest, very quickly, or be changed overnight by legislation. The practical implication of this difference in time-scale is that any government wishing to change the consumption patterns of its citizens – as British governments have wanted to do more than once in the last 250 years – has to manipulate availability, unless it is content to wait a decade or more for significant change to occur. It is important to appreciate, though, that demand and availability are interdependent. Commercial forces will ensure that any sustained increase or decrease in demand eventually leads to corresponding changes in availability, and any sustained change in availability will result in a change in attitudes to alcohol, and hence to changes in demand. And, of course, the political acceptability of legislation to alter availability, in either direction, will be influenced by the same cultural and religious traditions and attitudes as those determining demand, as well as by anxieties about the balance of trade, unemployment, and vested interests.

Factors influencing demand

Alcohol has innumerable roles and functions in our society and some of these have been referred to already in Chapter 2. Before the First World War, except in the highest and the lowest ranks of society, drinking was largely a male prerogative. This is, of course, no longer so but drinking, particularly beer drinking, is still to some extent a symbol of masculinity. One of the main reasons why adolescents start drinking is to demonstrate that they are grown up, and young men still seek to measure their manhood by the number of pints they can down in an evening. Because of these masculine connotations drinking alcohol, like smoking, is also to some extent a symbol of female emancipation. Girls start drinking in part to demonstrate that they are not to be outdone. Each year we read of tragic cases where a young person has died following an overdose of alcohol taken as a boast or dare.

There are still important differences in attitudes to alcohol and in the role alcohol plays in everyday life in different social classes and different parts of the British Isles, although they are much less important than they used to be, and are waning fast with increasing social and geographical mobility. The role of beer drinking as a symbol of masculinity is still more prominent in the north than the south, there are still far more teetotallers in Ireland, north and south, than in England, and women still drink far less than men. But Scottish bars have begun to acquire some of the comforts of the English pub, Sunday opening has spread to Wales, and women journalists now stand at the bar in El Vino's. International differences are fading equally rapidly, and for similar reasons. The French, particularly the young, have developed a taste for whisky and beer, African villagers drink bottled beer, and the British drink ever increasing quantities of lager and wine.

Although the emergence of new drinking patterns, and changes in the role of alcohol in different social situations, regions, and social groupings may all influence per capita consumption, their overall effect is, in the short term, less important than that of consumer purchasing power. Consumption almost invariably rises in times of increasing prosperity and falls when incomes fall. The way in which British per capita consumption rose steadily during the second half of the nineteenth century, and again between 1950 and the mid-1970s, has already been described. It fell sharply during the great depression in the early 1930s and again, though much less dramatically, between 1979 and 1982. Consumption also rose faster in the post-war years in countries like West Germany and the Netherlands, whose prosperity was increasing faster than ours. And as was pointed out in Chapter 2, these cyclical changes in demand resulting from periodic fluctuations in economic activity are generally amplified by cyclical changes in public attitudes.

Because consumption has risen in many countries in the last fifteen years to higher levels than at any time since before the First World War, public concern about contemporary drinking habits and their consequences has also been increasing. In this context many attempts have been made in the last ten years, by national and local governments and by private organizations, to reduce the steadily rising demand for alcoholic beverages either by imposing restrictions on advertising or by health education. So far there is little evidence that either technique has been effective. Health education campaigns can often be shown to have made their target audience better informed, and even to have altered their attitudes, but they have not yet been shown to alter actual drinking behaviour. This does not mean, of course, that health education might not have a profound effect if sufficient funds were provided to sustain a major campaign over ten or twenty years. The fact that at present we lack evidence that health education campaigns are effective does not mean that they are necessarily ineffective. But it does mean that enthusiasms for health education have to be treated with caution. The situation is very similar where advertising is concerned. A total lack of alcohol advertising in Poland and the USSR has not prevented consumption from rising alarmingly in both those countries. Nor has the French government's recent restriction on the advertising of whisky apparently prevented the French from drinking it in increasing amounts. It is true that alcohol consumption has fallen in

Norway and Sweden since their governments placed severe restrictions on advertising a few years ago, but the contribution of these restrictions to this reduction is still uncertain. On the other hand an econometric analysis of the demand for alcoholic beverages in the United Kingdom between 1956 and 1975 did suggest that the advertising of spirits (though not of beer or wines) had resulted in increased consumption, which implies that a reduction in spirits advertising would have led to a fall in consumption. On the whole, there is little convincing evidence at present to refute the alcohol and tobacco industries' oft repeated claim that advertising only affects brand preferences and not overall levels of consumption. As with health education, though, a lack of evidence that advertising increases overall consumption levels is not the same as proof that it does not. It is indeed rather difficult to believe that all those successful young women sipping exotic cocktails, and all those happy and healthy looking workmen downing their pints on so many TV screens and hoardings never persuade someone to have a drink they would not otherwise have had.

Factors influencing availability

Availability can be influenced in a wide variety of ways, many of which have been freely utilized by governments, in some cases for hundreds of years. Controls may be placed on the production or the importation of alcoholic beverages. These may take the form of controls on the crop from which the beverage is produced (vines or barley, for example) or direct controls on the volume of beverage produced or sold. This may be done either by regulating the industries concerned, or by taking them into government ownership. In Finland, for example, the production and importation of alcoholic beverages are entirely in the hands of a government agency, Alko, and in Ontario and several American states all liquor stores are state owned. Indeed, in 1915 Lloyd George's cabinet seriously considered bringing British public houses under government ownership and did indeed nationalize a few pubs at that time. Sometimes the failure of a vital crop means that availability is reduced without the government or anyone else having intended it. In Poland, for example, there was a very poor harvest in 1981 and as the Polish government was then too short of foreign currency to import grain from its neighbours the quantity of vodka produced that year was 30 per cent less than in 1980. Controls can be, and often are, imposed on the places and times at which alcoholic beverages can be purchased, or consumed – licensed premises and licensing hours. There may also be controls on the purchaser. In most industrial countries children are not allowed to buy alcoholic beverages and earlier this century some countries attempted, unsuccessfully, to deprive known drunkards of the right to purchase alcoholic drinks. Finally, there are often special taxes on alcoholic beverages. In Britain this has been the case for well over three hundred years, since 1643.

Although there is good evidence that these various controls may be highly effective, relatively little is known about the efficacy of individual measures because governments wishing either to reduce alcohol consumption or to allow it to rise have usually, and probably very wisely, introduced (or relaxed) several different kinds of control simultaneously. In Britain, for example, beer consumption was reduced by 63 per cent and spirits consumption by 52 per cent between 1914 and 1918 by a government determined to curb drunkenness in munitions factories. This was achieved mainly by reducing both the number of licensed premises and their opening hours, but at the same time controls were placed on the production of beer and spirits, their alcohol content was reduced, 'off sale' hours were reduced, and it was made illegal to sell liquor on credit. And, of course, a high proportion of the country's young men were simultaneously entering the armed forces and moving overseas. In the 1960s, several American states reduced their minimum drinking age from twenty or twenty-one to eighteen. This resulted in so alarming an increase in road traffic accidents involving juvenile drivers that by 1975 several of these states had decided to raise the minimum age once more. In the process they had learnt that, although the original age limit had undoubtedly been widely flouted, the law in question had none the less been effective in restricting dangerous teenage drinking.

Controls on outlets (licensed premises) may be very effective in restricting consumption if those outlets are few and far between. The creation of large numbers of new outlets in Finland from 1969 onwards was associated with a rapid rise in per capita consumption. Between 1968 and 1970 the number of shops, restaurants, and bars licensed to sell alcohol was allowed to increase thirteenfold and per capita consumption rose by 50 per cent during those two years. Whether the number of outlets has any significant influence on consumption levels beyond the point at which there are one or two in every neighbourhood is less certain. The econometric analysis of United Kingdom consumption referred to above suggested that the number of retail outlets ('on' and 'off' licences combined) had been an important determinant of consumption between 1956 and 1975 despite their very large numbers (there were 156,000 in 1975). It is also widely believed that the 1961 Licensing Act and the abolition of resale price maintenance in 1966/67, which encouraged grocery chains and supermarkets to start selling alcoholic drinks, played an important role in the rapid increase in female drinking and female alcohol problems that has taken place in the last twenty years. One might imagine that with about 180,000 licensed premises to choose from (the figure is only approximate because the Home Office gave up trying to count them after 1980) a few thousand more or less would be unlikely to have any significant effect on consumption. Econometric analysis suggests, however, that if there had been 1 per cent fewer (i.e. 1,600 fewer) licensed premises in the United Kingdom in 1975, per capita consumption that year would have been 2.15 per cent lower.

The influence of restricted opening hours and the likely effect of changes in these is also uncertain, and more contentious in view of current pressure from the tourist industry and the liquor trade for a relaxation of present English controls. The increase in Scottish opening hours that occurred in 1976 and 1977 in response to the recommendations of the Clayson report has not been followed by any increase in public drunkenness, and probably not by any increase in per capita consumption either. As is so often the case, however, it is difficult to be sure because other changes were taking place at the same time, in this case the onset of economic recession, falling disposable incomes, and a ban on police overtime in Strathclyde. On the whole the evidence suggests that severe restrictions on opening hours may have the harmful effect of encouraging rapid drinking to 'beat the clock', and that removing these restrictions may help to *reduce* public drunkenness and drunken driving. At the same time, however, it may *increase* total consumption and therefore increase other ill effects, such as cirrhosis.

In the absence of draconian controls of other kinds, price is the most effective regulator of alcohol consumption. There is abundant evidence from many different countries and time periods that consumption almost invariably rises when the real price of alcohol (i.e. the price relative to the price of other goods, or the cost of living index) falls, and falls when the real price rises. The quantity of beer consumed in England dropped sharply when the original (1643) duty was tripled in 1690, and again when the duty on malt was tripled in 1791. Conversely, the reduction in duty involved in the free mash tun system introduced by Gladstone in 1880, coupled with the nation's rising prosperity, caused beer consumption to rise to record levels at the end of the nineteenth century. Consumption of wines and spirits has been equally sensitive to changes in taxation. The 1751 act 'for more effectually restraining the retailing of distilled spirituous liquors' and the Disorderly Houses Act of 1752 produced a dramatic reduction in gin consumption. The Methuen Treaty of 1703, which allowed Portuguese wines to be imported cheaply, effectively persuaded the leisured classes to drink port rather than claret and consumption of French wines did not recover until the duty on them was reduced by the Cobden Treaty of 1860.

In the last ten years, detailed investigations have been made of the relationship between consumption and price in several different countries. Most of these have found a remarkably close relationship between the two. A group of Canadian research workers examined the relationship between per capita consumption of alcohol and the price of alcohol relative to personal disposable income in the Province of Ontario between 1928 and 1967. The two were virtually mirror images of one another. As the price of alcohol rose between 1929 and 1933 consumption fell steadily, but when the price started to fall, as it did progressively from 1934 to 1968, consumption rose higher and higher. A similar study was carried out for Denmark between 1915 and 1975. The investigators plotted total Danish consumption of different alcoholic beverages in litres per person per year against the quantity of that beverage obtainable by an average industrial employee working for 30 hours. For spirits the relationship was close; for beer it was almost perfect (see Figure 3). Consumption rose steadily as purchasing power increased, particularly from 1960 onwards, and every fluctuation in purchasing power was reflected in a corresponding change in consumption. In this country there has been a clear association between consumption and the cost of alcohol expressed as a percentage of mean per capita disposable income (see Figure 4).

The only well-documented instance of rising prices failing to result in reduced consumption is provided by Ireland, for Irish per capita consumption doubled between 1960 and 1974 despite a 21 per cent rise in the real price of alcohol between 1961 and 1970. This is not so anomalous as it appears at first sight, however. The period between 1960 and 1974 was one of steadily rising prosperity in Ireland and if beer and spirits prices had been calculated relative to personal disposable income they would almost certainly have been found to be falling rather than rising. Moreover, a high proportion of the Irish population used to be teetotallers and much of the rise in per capita consumption that occurred between 1960 and 1979 would have been due to the recruitment into the drinking population of young men and women whose parents were abstainers. Even so, this Irish evidence does draw attention to the fact that rising prices may have little or no effect on consumption if earnings are rising rapidly at the same time. If

Figure 3   *The relationship between the price of beer and consumer purchasing power in Denmark, 1915–75*

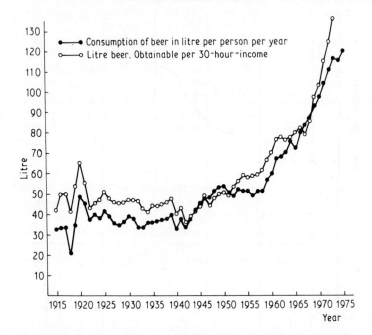

Source: Nielsen and Sorensen, Alcohol policy: alcohol consumption, alcohol prices, delirium tremens and alcoholism as cause of death in Denmark, *Social Psychiatry* 14: 133–38, 1979.

people can still afford to drink as much as before without having to reduce their expenditure on other things they may continue to do so. The crucial variable is price relative to average disposable income rather than the nominal price or even the 'real' (inflation adjusted) price.

It is often suggested, particularly by representatives of the alcohol industry, that although increasing the price of alcoholic beverages by increased taxation might indeed reduce per capita consumption, it would be a very inefficient means of reducing the ill effects of excessive consumption, because only 'normal social drinkers' would drink less. Alcoholics, so their argument goes, would be compelled by their addiction to drink as much as ever and their families might suffer

Figure 4   *Cost per pint of 100% alcohol as percentage of personal disposable income at current prices compared to annual consumption per head of population*

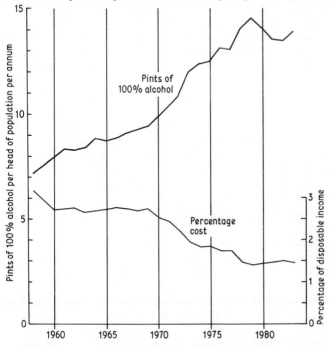

Source: Health Education – The Prevention of Alcohol-Related Problems, Scottish Health
    Education Co-ordinating Committee, 1985.

greater hardships than before as an even higher proportion of the
family income went on alcohol. Despite its superficial plausibility, this
argument is fallacious. Some of the reasons have been referred to
above, and in any case there are several well-documented examples of
a rise in liquor prices leading directly to a reduction in ill effects, and
this could hardly occur unless a significant proportion of those who
were previously drinking excessively did reduce their intake. In 1854,
for example, the excise duty on spirits was increased in Scotland to
bring it into line with England. Whisky consumption promptly fell by
13 per cent and this was accompanied by a 12 per cent fall in criminal
convictions in Scotland and a 25 per cent fall in offences against
property in Edinburgh. In 1917 the Danish government imposed a
crippling tax on what was then the Danes' main alcoholic drink, a

distilled spirit called akvavit, which cut consumption by nearly 80 per cent. Within a year hospital admissions for delirium tremens had fallen by no less than 93 per cent and deaths from chronic alcoholism by 86 per cent. More recently a West Indian psychiatrist, Professor Beaubrun, has shown that in Trinidad between 1966 and 1975 there was an almost perfect inverse relationship between the number of road traffic accidents each year and the price of rum (the island's main drink) relative to per capita income. Whenever the price of rum fell, accidents increased and when it rose, they decreased. A similar relationship has been demonstrated in the United States between changes in state liquor taxes between 1960 and 1974 and changes in cirrhosis mortality, increased taxation being associated with a reduction in cirrhosis mortality and decreased taxation with a rise in mortality. Finally, a recent Scottish study has provided us with information about the drinking habits of a representative group of 'regular drinkers' both before and after a price rise. The rise in question was mainly due to the increase in excise duty on beer and other alcoholic beverages in the March 1981 budget, which caused their price to rise faster than the retail price index or average disposable incomes for the first time in thirty years. Between 1978/79 and 1981/82, the average weekly alcohol consumption of the 463 people interviewed on both occasions fell by 18 per cent and their 'adverse effects' score by 16 per cent. Furthermore, those who had been heavy or dependent drinkers in 1978/79 reduced their consumption at least as much as light or moderate drinkers, and suffered fewer adverse effects as a result. This study thus provides direct evidence that heavy drinkers are influenced by increased prices just as much as more moderate drinkers, and benefit personally from their reduced consumption into the bargain.

In summary, therefore, a wide range of factors influence per capita consumption, by influencing either the demand for alcoholic beverages or their availability. Cultural traditions and consumer purchasing power are the most important determinants of demand but the former are slow to change and not easily manipulated. Availability can change, or be changed by legislation, much more rapidly. A wide variety of legislative controls on availability have been used in the past and many of these are currently in use, albeit in attenuated form, in this country. In the absence of draconian controls of other kinds the price of alcoholic beverages relative to disposable income is the most important determinant of per capita consumption, and the fall in this ratio in the United Kingdom between 1950 and the late 1970s was probably the main cause of the doubling of per capita consumption that took place during that period.

SOCIAL INFLUENCES ON INDIVIDUAL CONSUMPTION

Until now, we have been discussing social or environmental influences which affect everyone, and so are liable to influence the consumption of the population as a whole. There are, however, a number of other important social influences which only affect particular groups of people. As we have seen, occupation is probably the most important of these, for some jobs are associated with a very high risk of alcohol dependence and other alcohol-related disorders (Table 10). Brewery and distillery workers, publicans and restaurateurs, waiters and cooks are in constant contact with alcoholic beverages and, legitimately or illegitimately, have fairly ready access to drinks for themselves. To some extent such occupations attract people who are already heavy drinkers; they choose to work in a brewery rather than a factory because of the free drinks they expect to obtain. But others who were not originally heavy drinkers become so because alcohol is so readily available and most of their colleagues or work mates are drinking. Company directors and salesmen are two other high risk groups, partly because of the longstanding tradition of negotiating business deals over a drink, or what is sometimes euphemistically called a 'working lunch'. Table 10 shows the standardized mortality ratios for death from cirrhosis of the liver for a number of high risk occupations. As cirrhosis mortality provides an indirect indication of a group's alcohol consumption this table probably provides a good index of the drinking habits of different occupations. As well as the obvious one of ready access to free or cheap liquor the important underlying risk factors are frequent absences from home, long and irregular working hours, high income, and lack of supervision.

The ethnic grouping to which an individual belongs is another potent determinant of his or her drinking habits. Social scientists have long been fascinated, for example, by the tendency of Irish communities throughout the English-speaking world to generate more drunkenness and more alcohol dependence than their neighbours, while Jewish communities almost invariably do the reverse. Why this should be so is much debated but part of the explanation probably lies in the different roles alcohol fulfils in these two cultures. Jewish families drink wine at home every week in a domestic religious setting. The Irish rarely drink at home or with their families. Instead men drink on their own in bars and male drunkenness is tolerated by the community. (It should be noted, though, that the per capita consumption of Ireland is no higher than that of the United Kingdom, partly because a relatively high proportion of the Irish are teetotallers.) It is also widely believed that

Table 10   *Standardized mortality ratios of different occupations for cirrhosis of the liver, England and Wales, 1970–72*

	Standardized mortality ratio
average occupation	100
publicans, innkeepers	1576
deck, engineering officers and pilots, ships	781
barmen, barmaids	633
deck and engine-room ratings, barge and boatmen	628
fishermen	595
proprietors and managers, boarding houses and hotels	506
finance, insurance brokers, financial agents	392
restauranteurs	385
lorry drivers' mates, van guards	377
armed forces (British and foreign)	367
cooks	354
shunters, pointsmen	323
winders, reelers	319
electrical engineers	316
authors, journalists, and related workers	314
medical practitioners	311

Note: By definition the average standardized mortality ratio is 100, so barmen and barmaids, for example, have a cirrhosis mortality more than six times the average.
Source: Office of Population Censuses and Surveys, 1978.

the Scots drink more, and more unwisely, than the English. It is certainly true that Scotland has more cirrhosis deaths and more hospital admissions for alcohol dependence than England and Wales, but when random samples of the population are surveyed and questioned about their drinking habits these appear to be remarkably similar in the two countries. Whether this is because the Scots really do drink no more than the English, or are merely more reluctant to admit how much they consume, is still uncertain and also much debated.

To some extent the very different drinking habits of men, women, and children are culturally transmitted in the same ways as the distinctive drinking habits of different ethnic groups. In most societies the situations in which men and women are allowed to drink, and sometimes expected to drink, are quite different. So too are the kinds of drinks they are expected to consume, and the quantity, and even the ways in which they are expected to behave when intoxicated. The 'unwritten rules' provided by these detailed cultural expectations are powerful determinants of people's actual behaviour, and are often more effective in restraining disruptive and antisocial behaviour than formal laws or regulations. It is often suggested, for example, that the lack of any established norms governing its use was an important part of the reason why the new drink gin caused such havoc in eighteenth century England, and why Western-style bottled beer is currently causing similar havoc in parts of Africa. Potent though they may be, however, the unwritten rules provided by these cultural expectations are not immutable. Those governing women's drinking in our society, for example, have changed dramatically within the last two generations. Recently there has been a disproportionate increase in alcohol consumption by young women. Surveys suggest that fifteen- and sixteen-year-old schoolgirls now drink almost as frequently as schoolboys of that age, and more than their grandmothers did at any age.

The amount people drink is also influenced by the 'stress' they are under. Although stress is a rather vague concept, and what is stressful to one person may not be so to someone else in an almost identical situation, it is a commonplace observation that somone who is anxious or worried, or in a situation of some kind which they are having difficulty coping with or adjusting to, often increases their intake of alcohol, sometimes with disastrous consequences. A man worried about the profitability of his business, or impending lay-offs in his industry, a husband distressed by his wife's increasing estrangement or the bad company his son is keeping, a wife lonely in a new city or worried about her health – all may start to drink more under these circumstances, and perhaps continue to do so when the anxieties or problems in question have been resolved. Often, of course, such periods of increased drinking may be short-lived and eminently understandable. But they are always rather ominous, because they are evidence that the individual concerned is starting to use alcohol as a drug, for its pharmacological effects rather than for its taste or its social concomitants. In those who eventually become dependent on alcohol it is frequently possible to identify a time of stress, often many years before, when they first began to drink more than other people. This sequence of events suggests, of course, that they might have been in some way more vulnerable than others. The elusive nature of this individual vulnerability will be discussed in the next chapter.

8

Individual causes of harmful drinking

Current evidence strongly supports the view that many interacting social influences play a part in harmful drinking. Does this mean, therefore, that we can safely ignore the possible role of individual characteristics, such as our genetic background or our personalities? On the contrary, what needs to be stressed is the complementary nature of the social and personal explanations. In discussing individual factors, what has to be borne in mind is that the individual with all his personal propensities lives in a social setting which will greatly determine which propensities are in fact developed.

Genetic causes

A common observation is that people with serious drinking problems quite often have a parent, brother, sister, or other relative who has experienced the same sort of problem. According to recent United States studies, about one-third of fathers, sons, husbands, or brothers of an alcohol dependent are likely to have a drinking problem and this is a much higher rate than would be expected by chance. Put simply, alcohol-related problems run in families, particularly in the males of the family.

Two different types of explanation could be offered for this observation. The popular one is the postulate which suggests that parental example is a potent influence – the problem drinker's son becomes a problem drinker much as the architect's son or daughter takes up the father's profession. A piece of research which has often been quoted as supporting this family environment type of explanation is a study published over forty years ago by Dr Ann Roe. She went through the records of a child fostering agency in New York and was able to find thirty-six cases where the biological father was an excessive drinker, and the child had been taken out of the original home before the age of ten years. A control group of fostered children from homes where there was no record of excessive drinking was also studied. The follow-up to an age of about thirty showed that there was no difference between these two fostered groups in adult drinking behaviour.

The alternative explanation for the drinking problem of the alcoholic child is genetic. The great bulk of evidence relating to social influences on drinking has frequently been interpreted as suggesting that there can be little room left for genetic explanations. However, there is no good reason to consider socio-cultural and genetic explanations as mutually exclusive and opposed. The past ten years has seen a resurgence of interest in human genetic studies of drinking and so much careful research has now been published on this topic that it cannot be safely ignored.

There have been four well-executed *twin studies* of problem drinking. In each of these, identical twins showed a greater similarity of drinking behaviour (concordance), and in some studies greater concordance for alcohol abuse, than did non-identical twins, who in theory shared the same family environment but not the same genes. The best designed *adoption studies* in this field were conducted by a team of American and Danish researchers. These also strongly support the argument for a genetic element. These studies involved interviewing the sons (average age thirty years) of Danish diagnosed 'alcoholics' raised by non-alcoholic parents, and a group of sons (average age thirty-three years) raised by their own alcoholic, biological parents. Paired with each of these two groups was a control group without alcoholic parents, matched for age and, in the adopted group, matched for circumstances of adoption. Ratings of alcoholism were made by psychiatrists blind to the hypothesis of the study and to the parentage of the subjects. Those men whose biological parents were diagnosed alcoholic were *four times more likely* to be alcoholic than were the sons of non-alcoholic biological parents. However, there was no significant relationship between alcohol abuse in adoptees and the presence or absence of alcohol abuse in their adoptive parents. In another study which involved the fostering of half-siblings, children with an alcoholic, biological parent who were raised by non-alcoholic parents had a rate of alcohol abuse *three times higher* than children without alcoholic parents who were raised by an alcoholic step-parent or surrogate.

This is not to suggest that a family environment where a parent is an alcoholic has no effect on whether a child will subsequently develop a drinking problem. In a large follow-up study of over 500 Boston boys, it was shown that about one in ten of those who grew up in households where neither parent nor parent surrogate abused alcohol subsequently became alcohol dependent compared with one in four of those reared by alcohol-abusing fathers and one in three reared by alcohol-abusing mothers.

Summarizing these research results, it does appear that while family atmosphere and influence contribute to the development of alcohol problems in later life, a significant fraction of the association between alcohol abuse in parents and in children is genetically rather than environmentally transmitted.

However, genetic studies of drinking and excessive drinking should be placed in a context of understanding provided by the larger background of general genetic research. It is common to find that *some* genetic contribution can be established for many aspects of human attributes or disorders (ranging from musical ability to premature balding) and drinking is unlikely to be an exception. What is much more difficult to establish is the precise degree of genetic contribution, the manner in which the genetic influence acts, and the extent to which genetic predisposition may be modified by environment.

The role of personality

One important cause put forward to explain why people drink excessively is that their personality in some way predisposes them to do so. To take an example, an ambitious woman who was striving and successful, but who despite outward appearances was lacking in social confidence, saw the origins of her drinking thus:

'I suppose I first discovered that a drink would do something for me pretty early on. At seventeen or eighteen I was quite desperately shy and it would be a real pain for me to have to go out to parties or out on a date, or join in any sort of social gathering. But then I found that if I could get a couple of drinks down, I'd be much less tense, really able to join the gang. For a good few years I just used drink that way, as a tranquillizer to get me through social situations. Then, when I was about thirty, my career began to go well and I got promotion, and was working very hard, and the job itself began to mean a lot of socializing; I didn't want to say "I can't do it, don't give me that promotion". That's when my drinking began to take off.'

The expectation that personality can be one of the determinants of excessive drinking derives support from a variety of research findings. One important line of research has been the community sample survey, which employs door-to-door interviews and which can provide information on the relationships between the quantity drunk, reasons given for drinking, problems with drinking and aspects of personality. A consistent finding is that heavier drinkers (and by implication people who have more problems with drinking) tend to be found among those using alcohol for 'personal' reasons. By this is meant the use of alcohol for the specific purpose of relieving 'bad nerves' or tension, or restlessness, or boredom, or as something that helps people to forget their worries. Thus the suggestion is that vulnerable personalities will find alcohol functionally useful as a nerve drug, which in turn will lead to heavy drinking and consequently to troubles with drinking. As one alcohol dependent patient explained 'alcohol anaesthetizes my feelings so that I can cope with life'.

But are we right in supposing that certain personalities are predisposed to harmful drinking or is the contrary explanation the correct one, that excessive drinking is itself the cause of the abnormalities detected by these personality tests? Heavy drinking can certainly result in 'bad nerves' (see p. 58). The obvious way to meet this difficulty is to set up studies which follow a large sample of children forward into adult life, and which could thereby determine whether any identifiable personality characteristics are predictive of the development of later drinking problems. Such an approach should also be able to identify any predictive features in the early home environment and family constellation which are associated with later risk of dependence.

In 1983, the results of what has been termed the biggest and most expensive behavioural science follow-up ever conducted were published. The study involved 500 men who were first studied in 1940, when they were aged between 11 and 16 years, by researchers at the Harvard Law School, and 200 men who were first studied in 1938 when they were Harvard undergraduates. This research involved a prodigious amount of record analysis, including personality test results, school and court reports, military records, academic performance, marital and family patterns, and various indicators of physical and mental health. Its author, Harvard psychiatrist George Vaillant, found that analysing the premorbid personalities of those children who subsequently developed alcohol problems did not reveal any trait or tendency which significantly distinguished them from those who did not subsequently misuse alcohol. If anything, those who became problem drinkers or alcohol dependent were more self-confident, more assertive and less anxious. In so far as any factors predicted alcohol abuse in adult life it was a family history of alcohol problems, ethnicity (Irish, Polish and Russo-Americans had high rates), and behaviour problems in adolescence.

These results do not provide support for the view that there is a particular 'alcoholic personality' which predisposes those who possess it to develop abnormal drinking patterns. On the contrary, there appear to be a great many personality traits which, given the right circumstances, predispose to excessive drinking and any of these traits can be found in varying degree rather than as absolutely present or absent. None of these personality characteristics is unique to people with drinking problems. In so far as Vaillant found a relationship between personality disturbances and alcohol misuse it was that alcohol contributed to the personality problem rather than the other way round, adding support to the Old Japanese proverb: 'First, the man takes a drink, then the drink takes a drink, then the drink takes the man.'

The range of ideas that psychology and psychiatry offer for understanding the individual alcohol abuser include explanations in terms of immaturity and impulsiveness of personality, defect in self-esteem, or dependence conflict. Excessive drinking has also been seen in some circumstances as a hostile or revengeful act in a person with strong aggressive tendencies, or as a more or less purposeful act of 'chronic suicide'. Others use a drink to achieve a sense of acute excitement – a 'high' state – not otherwise available to them. Alcohol may be taken to anaesthetize feelings or inner conflicts. For instance, Baudelaire, writing about Edgar Allan Poe, observed that 'he drank . . . as if he were performing a homicidal function, as if he had to kill something inside himself, a worm that would not die.'

To take one clinical example in a little more detail, the excessive drinker who lacks self-confidence, has little self-esteem, and may even be disgusted with themselves, can sometimes be very readily identified. Often such a person will have been deprived of affection in childhood, sometimes frankly neglected, or even brutally or sexually mistreated. Patients describe cold, unloving parents who expected the worst of them, and constantly criticized their offspring. Such individuals may then use alcohol as a respite from mental self-flagellation and from a pervading sense of insufficiency and inferiority which often long predates the onset of dependence.

A second example is of a very different type of person quite free from self-loathing and not troubled in personal relationships. This is the self-indulgent individual who was pampered in childhood by doting or anxious parents. He or she may have been the only child or the youngster for whom everything was done and on whom few demands were imposed, or the sheltered being who never really needed to fend for him/herself. Such a person can find the harsh realities of work, personal relations, and marriage add up to a bleak vista of obligations and responsibilities. Such personalities may meet these responsibilities more or less effectively but may also discover that drinking can confer a mental holiday. When under the influence of alcohol to the right extent, exciting reveries can be summoned to transform mundane existence. In treatment, the hedonistic patient who has been seeking euphoria seems to do rather better than the self-punitive alcohol dependent who lets up on himself or herself only when drinking.

These two types of drinker have been described to illustrate how differently the personality can be organized before heavy drinking develops. Listening to people who themselves have tried to understand what it was in their personalities that predisposed to heavy drinking suggests that there is indeed a range of modestly useful generalizations. However, such retrospective analyses remain confounded by the very real possibility that the traits, tendencies, vulnerabilities, and difficulties identified by the drinker and his doctor as possible causes or contributors to the problem of alcohol misuse may in fact be more accurately interpreted as the result. The more an individual misuses alcohol the more maladjusted and psychologically impaired he or she will appear to be.

Psychiatric illness as an individual predisposing factor

In the preceding section we have looked at the ways in which personality may predispose to excessive drinking. By 'personality' is meant the sort of person, the cast of temperament, the sum of psychological attributes – the variations on the normal themes of human character. Less common than personality predisposition or variation in psychological constitution are those instances where discreet and diagnosable mental illness underlies the development of a drinking problem. If some of these illnesses were more adequately treated (or after-care more effectively organized), a contribution might be made to the prevention of drinking problems, and in some instances an underlying mental illness might point to the type of treatment that may be needed.

Perhaps the most common association is with depressive illness. By depressive illness we mean not the tendency on occasion to feel a bit down in the dumps, which is in different degrees part of everyone's experience and for some people a major and life-long temperamental problem associated with other difficulties in adjustment, but the definitely recognizable mental illness often developing in the previously normal person. It can be a response to stress, bereavement, the menopause, retirement, or it can be quite unheralded. The person suffering from this illness may not fully realize what is happening but engage in self-blame. A woman described her experience thus:

> 'I nursed my mother for about two years. Up every night, but never any difficulty in keeping going. When she died everyone said how sensibly I took it. But six months later it caught up with me – just couldn't stop crying, wanted to shut myself away, felt just so ill. I'd had a bottle of brandy in the house for my mother, and I thought, well, it might be a bit of a pick-me-up. I don't think anything happened suddenly, she died eighteen months ago, and, well, I suppose now I'm getting through half a bottle some days, it doesn't really do any good, but to begin with . . .'

The familiar story is often indeed of a grieving woman or man who has sought to alleviate this misery with drinking. In the short term, alcohol can be potent in giving relief. But it is in fact not an anti-depressant. It will, in many respects, make the condition worse, although it may continue to give a transient and superficial relief which encourages its continuing heavy use. The woman described above recovered rapidly when she received counselling concerning her loss coupled with judicious use of anti-depressant medication.

It is important to recognize that the life of the problem drinker is inherently depressing – waking with a hangover, feeling guilty about misdemeanours when drunk, and full of remorse at being unable to drink more sensibly. It is little wonder that many complain of depression. This more common form of lowering of mood often improves dramatically after a few days of abstinence and does not require any specific drug treatment.

Another quite common underlying psychiatric condition is the severe anxiety state; or some form of situational anxiety, such as agoraphobia or claustrophobia. Phobic conditions are often treatable, so that diagnosis is of practical importance. Excessive drinking can sometimes be a consequence of loss of psychological control resulting from organic damage to the brain. The old person who is suffering from dementia can begin to drink in a dangerous manner, or the young person who, for example, has sustained a severe head injury in a motor cycle accident may a year later be drinking in a disastrously chaotic fashion. Rarely, excessive drinking may be a complication of mental subnormality.

More unusual mental causes include schizophrenia, and particularly that type of the illness which has as its end result the person who is psychologically withdrawn, emotionally flattened, and quietly listening to his 'voices', while socially he or she is homeless, drifting, unable to work, and falling through the systems of social after-care – drink is added as one more problem. Occasionally, too, the person who has periods of abnormal elation (hypomania) will drink excessively in the phase of excitement. This is partly perhaps because of the general impairment of judgement and responsibility and sense of free-spending expansiveness that is typical of this disorder, and partly too because the elation may in fact be accompanied by much anxiety, or rather superficially masked depression.

What can, therefore, be concluded from this brief review of the possible relationship between mental illness and drinking is that, although mental illness only makes a relatively small contribution to the genesis of abnormal drinking, the possibilities should be borne in mind. To neglect an underlying mental illness may be harmful, while to treat that illness may be the key to helping with the drinking problem.

THE MAJOR IMPLICATIONS

These last two chapters can be rounded off by making or reiterating two very simple and definite points. The first is that there is a vast and growing amount of research and observations from many different scientific and clinical disciplines which today bear on the understanding of why people drink harmfully. This mass of information is a challenge in its own right. It can be left on the library shelves and quietly ignored while government policies and the daily business of all our dealings go ahead on the basis of uninformed predilections. Alternatively, this or that piece of evidence can be taken out of context, accorded dominant importance, and all reservations in interpretation forgotten; price control becomes everything, genetics takes the centre of the stage or gets entirely rejected, early environment is the whole explanation. Different scientific disciplines will each put in their bid and if the scientists fail to understand each other it is hardly surprising that the lay man is left in a muddle. It is often extraordinarily difficult to establish the satisfactory and sensible follow-through from even a relatively straightforward piece of research to social action and policies. In this particular instance the complexities and difficulties are such that there is a very live risk of getting lost in a fog. The abolition of the Royal Navy's daily rum ration was recommended in 1834 and implemented in 1968.

The second essential point is that we do not have to end up in a fog. Rather, the aim, endorsed in the very idea of a report such as this, is to enable as many people as possible, from the general public to the professionals and politicians, to examine closely the whole range of evidence so that we may be able to take from it *any understanding that offers a way to tackle effectively the problems concerned.* There is a heavy responsibility on us all to identify ways whereby society can both reduce the appalling rates of alcohol-related damage and treat the many people who are suffering.

9

Choice and personal responsibility

The ultimate choice about when and how much to drink, or whether to drink alcohol at all, lies with the individual. This chapter is concerned with the responsibility of the individual for his or her own drinking. It also discusses our responsibility as parents, friends, hosts or hostesses, and participants in the life of the community.

INDIVIDUAL RESPONSIBILITIES

There are a number of considerations which need to be made about our individual drinking choices. The pressure to drink is much greater on some than others but there is nothing inevitable about a particular drinking career. Choices exist at every stage. The points discussed below are not a list of taboos to be reluctantly obeyed, rather they consist of guidelines which may help all those who drink alcohol to become a little more conscious of their own drinking and its likely consequences.

Terms such as 'drinking too much' and 'needing to cut down' are impossibly vague and allow too much scope for self-deception. What is excess for a puritan may be regarded as moderation by a more indulgent character. Fortunately the concept of 'units of alcohol' discussed elsewhere in this book (pp. 43–4) provides a simple guide to measurement which has brought some clarity to the debate about sensible drinking. Familiarity with these units provides a ready means of calculating the quantity of alcohol consumed per occasion whatever the actual beverage choice. Table 11 shows how much alcohol is found in different drinks and translates these differences into the approximate number of units of alcohol which are found in conventional measures. The drinker should, however, bear in mind that the measures which

Table 11   *Conversion of volumes of alcohol beverages to grams of alcohol*

beverage	alcohol g/100 ml	alcohol in standard measure	
brown ale bottle	2.2	12.4 g/pint	
canned bitter	3.1	13.2 g/15 oz can	
draught bitter	3.1	17.6 g/pint	
draught mild	2.6	14.7 g/pint	
lager bottled	3.2	13.5 g/15 oz bottle	
stout extra	4.3	18.3 g/15 oz bottle	
strong ale, special lagers	6.6	28.0 g/15 oz bottle	
cider	3.8	21.5 g/pint	29.6 g/bottle
cider vintage	10.5	50.0 g/pint	82.0 g/bottle
red wine	9.5	11 g/glass	71.0 g/bottle
rosé	8.7	10 g/glass	65.0 g/bottle
white wine, dry	9.1	10 g/glass	64.0 g/bottle
white wine, medium	8.8	10 g/glass	62.0 g/bottle
white wine, sweet	10.2	11 g/glass	71.0 g/bottle
white wine, sparkling	9.9	11 g/glass	74.0 g/bottle
port	15.9	124 g/bottle	
sherry, dry	15.7	123 g/bottle	
sherry, medium	14.8	115 g/bottle	
sherry, sweet	15.6	122 g/bottle	
vermouth, dry	13.9	122 g/bottle	
advocaat	12.8	100 g/bottle	
cherry brandy	19.0	148 g/bottle	
Curacao	29.3	229 g/bottle	
spirts 70% (brandy, gin, whisky)	31.7	240 g/bottle	7.5 g/single measure

Note: 8g alcohol is one unit or standard drink which is approximately equal to the alcohol contained in 1 single measure of spirits / 1 glass of wine / ½ pint of beer (see Figure 1, p. 42)

are served at home or at parties are commonly far in excess of those dispensed by publicans!

Evidence suggests that the potential for personal harm increases greatly above the following limits:

50 units of alcohol per week for men (400g alcohol)
35 units of alcohol per week for women (280g alcohol)

If an individual chooses to be a regular drinker, then it is sensible to remain well below these limits. A moment's thought will show that these guidelines must not be taken too literally and are inadequate for certain circumstances. For example, driving while under the influence of any alcohol is potentially dangerous. On average, it takes one hour for the body to get rid of one standard drink (8g alcohol) although it should be borne in mind that wide individual variation exists here and the factors mentioned on p. 43 influence absorption. It is important to know enough about alcohol to be able to calculate when it is likely to be completely out of the system before driving or engaging in any other complex or hazardous pursuit. It is quite common for someone to drink 20 units of alcohol at a party and as a consequence prove a danger on the roads or at work the next morning when their blood alcohol level is still well above 80mg. The reader will recall that many accidents at home and at work are the result of intoxication or a hangover. Table 12 shows the effect of various levels of alcohol consumption and some of their likely consequences. If we are going to use the drug alcohol, it is in our own interests and those of others that we should know about the drug and its effects at different dosages.

Because of differences in body weight and in the distribution of water and fat within the body, the sex and size of the drinker are important considerations. Women have a lower ceiling for harm-free drinking than men. As mentioned in Chapter 6, only minimal drinking is advisable during pregnancy.

Guidelines to sensible drinking must be approached with common sense. If one week's consumption is made up of a single binge consuming twelve pints of beer, then the consequences in terms of sickness, drunkenness, and accidents may prove very serious and yet the average weekly consumption of units may not be disturbingly high. The pattern of drinking – where, when, how much, and how often – is just as important as the weekly count of units. Regular daily drinking is more likely to lead to liver damage and dependence; quite regular drinking may cause no concern to anyone, until after a period of twenty years or so cirrhosis of the liver or cancer of the gullet develops. Spree or bout drinking interspersed with sobriety more often gives rise to various forms of social harm and accidents when intoxicated. The following hints concerning sensible drinking are useful guidelines for all drinkers:

Table 12 *Behaviour and blood alcohol concentration*

Blood alcohol concentration (mg%)	Typical effects for an individual of average alcohol tolerance
20	enhanced sense of well-being visual reaction time reduced
40	somewhat disinhibited reduced driving ability at speed
60	judgement impaired
80	physical co-ordination impaired
100	evident loss of social judgement and poorly co-ordinated
130	clearly intoxicated
300	coma, stupor, loss of bladder control
500+	coma, respiratory depression, death

1. Don't drink every day of the week – try to introduce two or three alcohol-free days. This gives the body a chance to recover.
2. Don't use alcohol as a means of helping you cope with emotional problems.
3. Don't drink alone.
4. Don't use alcohol as a nightcap to help you sleep. You will quickly become tolerant of this regular dose and then find that you have to increase it to obtain a satisfactory result.
5. Don't drink alcohol while taking other drugs, either prescribed or 'over the counter'.
6. Don't drink on an empty stomach. Try to have something to eat while you are drinking. This delays absorption of alcohol.
7. If you are participating in a drinking session try to introduce a non-alcoholic drink into your drinking sequence. It is often a good idea to quench thirst first with a non-alcoholic drink.
8. Always put your glass down between sips and try to pace your drinking so that you become one of the slower drinkers in company.

9. Sip, don't gulp your drinks.

10. If you drink spirits, always dilute them.

In what circumstances should individuals become concerned about their drinking? It is worthwhile for all drinkers from time to time to take stock of their drinking by making a note of what has been consumed in a week and adding up the total units. If this total regularly exceeds the guidelines, then it is definitely time to reduce. Total units are not the only pointer. An excessive drinker when asked when he knew that alcohol was a problem announced: 'I knew when alcohol began to cost me more than just money.'

Individuals will have different reasons for reducing consumption. It may be costing too much so that other aspects of the family budget are suffering; causing accidents or inefficiency at work; causing hangovers, weight gain, or ill health; or family and friends may be upset. An individual may simply decide that too great a part of their time and recreation is being devoted to drinking and that a change toward a more varied life-style is desirable. There are many other factors which may help someone decide that they really should take some positive steps to cut down their drinking. For most people there is some 'last straw' which changes a vague ambition into a definitive resolve to take action, for example:

Tony was twenty-five. He had been a regular social drinker ever since he was seventeen. He drank a lot with his friends during his apprenticeship and even after he got married he continued the habit of going out two or three evenings a week with those of his friends who would still join him. He never liked to give up that adolescent style of life even when his wife asked him to cut back. He felt that to change would be to admit that he was being dominated by his wife and that he was getting old like his father – 'reduced' to sitting in front of the TV. He also drank a lot at weekends when he would drink before the football match and in the evenings he and his wife would go to parties. He frequently had bad hangovers in the mornings. He often promised himself and his wife that he would cut down but he never did this for more than a few days. One morning, while dressing, he looked in the mirror and seeing his bloodshot, baggy eyes and his flabby paunch, he thought he looked middle aged. He also felt sick but could not take any more time off work. He knew he was not as sharp as he used to be at his trade; he was not the kind of person he really wanted to be. On this occasion he resolved on his own with no one else present to make a real change in his drinking habits. For him the prematurely ageing face in the mirror was the 'last straw' and he became motivated to change.

Lisa was twenty-five. She had been married for six years and had two children, one aged eighteen months and Lucy aged five. Her husband made quite a lot of money working on the oil rigs but he was rarely at home. She felt isolated and the children got on her nerves. She felt guilty about this. When her husband was away, she had got into the habit of fortifying herself for the day's chores by drinking Martini. Usually she drank about three generous measures each afternoon but when she was tense or the children particularly trying, she might drink as much as a bottle, then she would feel sick and guilty. Her mother and her husband had both asked her to stop and a health visitor had warned her about drinking too much. These pieces of advice had made her feel more guilty and angry, with them and with herself. One day she fell asleep in the afternoon and accidentally burned a hole in the couch with her lighted cigarette. She woke in a frightful state and quickly put it out. She ran around the house screaming and crying. Seeing the state she was in, Lucy said, 'Shall I get you your drink from the fridge?' For Lisa this was the 'last straw'. She was not too upset at setting fire to the couch, which had happened before, but she was deeply distressed by the fact that her daughter knew her so well and knew what an important part drinking played in her life. Following that experience, she resolved to change her habits and succeeded.

Resolutions of this kind have often been contemplated and attempted many times before but there is commonly some experience which tilts the balance in favour of making a real change. It is never easy for any of us to change a well-established habit. Most people will have had the experience of making resolutions which they fail to keep. Resolving to change a habit and maintaining that resolve is obviously more difficult the more socially, psychologically, and sometimes physically important that habit has become. The reader will realize from earlier chapters that changing a drinking habit can be extremely difficult and may require some form of outside help (Chapter 10). There are, none the less, many people who, on their own, succeed in reducing their alcohol consumption to safer levels. The first phase is recognizing that a problem exists, the next is resolving to take action: having resolved to take action various 'self-help' techniques are available which an individual may use as tools towards achieving the desired goal. There are also a number of self-help manuals available which provide structure and guidance about the task ahead (see bibliography, p. 191).

Taking stock

It is often helpful to take stock of the nature of the problem which alcohol is causing before working out means of dealing with it. A balance sheet (see the example in Figure 5) can be drawn up enumerating the advantages and disadvantages of a particular course of action. It need not, of course, be as formal as this but it seems helpful to set some objectives down on paper and acknowledge some of the gains and losses which are likely to follow a change in drinking patterns.

Figure 5   *Balance Sheet*

Example drawn up by George, aged 30, based on self-help manual

action	advantages	disadvantages
making no change	keep up with my drinking friends	it is costing me too much
	forget my worries	it really adds to my worries next day
	show Jane (wife) she can't dominate me	
drinking less	save money	
	fewer rows at home	I would have to explain to my friends
	fewer hangovers	I will miss the good feeling drinking brings when I am tired and depressed
	more efficient at work	
	lose weight	

Setting goals

It is preferable to set a realistic and attainable goal, such as drinking only two pints in the evening and cutting out one evening in the pub each week, rather than being overambitious at first and failing. Having agreed on an objective, it often helps if the plan can be discussed with a close relative or friend. This other person can provide support and encouragement as well as a critical reminder about the ease with which we can delude ourselves that progress is being made despite all evidence to the contrary. Self-help techniques are most relevant for those who are beginning to drink in a hazardous way and wish to return to a more sensible pattern. For those who are very dependent on alcohol, any attempt to cut down may prove difficult because withdrawal symptoms develop (see Chapter 6). In such circumstances it is best to seek professional help.

Self-monitoring

A regular diary is a most useful tool in assessing the nature of a drinking habit and in monitoring progress towards the set goal. First, a diary may be used to obtain an objective measure of weekly consumption and the pattern of drinking (see Figure 6). This pattern provides pointers to the difficult times of the week when past experience suggests that most drink is likely to be taken. These 'at risk' times will need particular attention in the plan. Second, the diary can then be used as a regular means of evaluating progress, first on a weekly basis and then more intermittently to ensure that targets are being achieved and maintained. The first steps can be quite small but many individuals find that they progress from these toward quite significant changes in life-style with the development of a range of new activities, interests, and values.

The balance sheet and diary can form a basis for self-monitoring. The balance sheet and diary shown in Figures 5 and 6 refer to George, aged thirty, and can be used as an example of the way in which an individual developed a self-help strategy. On the basis of the evidence shown George decided that he would reduce his alcohol intake to drinking on not more than four days weekly and not more than three pints or its equivalent on any one occasion. He estimated that he would make considerable financial savings by this strategy, see more of his family, improve relations with his wife, and yet maintain some contact with his friends. Looking at his diary, he agreed it was a fairly typical week and that there were a number of particular difficulties he would have to overcome to achieve his goal. The most conspicuous of these was his regular evening drinking session on the way home. He overcame this by telling his friends what he was trying to do and that he would meet them only on Monday and Friday as he now intended to be

Figure 6   *Sample diary prepared by George*

day	occasion	alcohol consumed	units	daily total
Monday	at pub on way home with friends	4 pints beer	8	8
Tuesday	at pub on way home with friends	2 pints beer	4	4
Wednesday	business lunch	2 large gins + tonic	4	
		½ bottle wine	4	
	at pub on way home with friends	3 pints beer	6	
	at home after dinner: row with wife about forgetting to collect daughter	3 large whiskies	9	23
Thursday	lunch alone in pub	2 double gins	4	
	at pub on way home with friends	2 pints beer	4	8
Friday	at pub on way home with friends	3 pints beer	6	
	dinner with wife and	1 bottle wine	8	
	two friends at home	1 whisky (double)	4	18
Saturday	lunchtime drink with friends	3 pints beer	6	
		2 whiskies (single)	2	
	drink with friends after football	2 pints beer	4	
	party with wife in evening	8 cans beer	12	24
Sunday	lunch at home	2 cans beer	3	3
		week's total units		88

at home earlier in the evening to help his daughter with her exam work. He stopped drinking at business lunches, stating to customers that alcohol made him too tired to concentrate in the afternoon. As it was their affairs he was looking after at that time, the customers seemed pleased by his responsible attitude. He continued to drink with his wife on a Friday night and to meet friends at lunchtime on Saturday. This goal was largely achieved over the course of two weeks. Thereafter, there were occasions when he went well outside his self-imposed limit, for instance at parties. He decided to accept these occasional sprees as harmless provided he returned to his general strategy the following day.

His relationship with his wife improved, although less than he had hoped, and he had more time with his son and daughter and found this very rewarding. He lost some friends who tended to leave him out of plans they made for fishing trips and football matches. He did, however, have time to renew a former interest in politics and become active in local party meetings. Although there were plenty of drinking occasions around these meetings, he had established himself in this new group as someone who rarely drank and he was accepted without difficulty on this basis.

This case example illustrates the way in which an individual can change habits provided he or she has the motivation coupled with a workable plan of action. Regular drinkers often find that they feel quite lost after giving up or reducing alcohol consumption. They may experience episodes of craving and longings but can be reassured that these will gradually pass. It is important to find alternative means of relaxing and coping with boredom or stress. Some helpful techniques, such as relaxation, can be learned. Various diversions, such as cooking, having a warm bath, or listening to music can help assuage feelings of craving. It is often a relief to learn that each episode of craving is usually quite short-lived, although they may of course recur. It is useful to have a list of alternative pursuits in mind as diversions to employ when the craving is most intense. Some helpful guide books now exist to assist this self-help process. They are listed in the bibliography.

There will be occasions when resolution fails and the goals are not achieved. A setback should not be taken as meaning that all is lost. It is important, however, to analyse the precipitants to the loss of resolve and to learn from the experience. Some drinkers may find that physical dependence or psychological difficulties or social pressures may make the task too difficult without help, and for some of these abstinence may prove the only workable goal (see Chapter 10). None the less, the majority of problem drinkers will have tried to make changes on their own long before they seek help and many succeed. Clinics and other agencies draw their clients from among those who for various reasons found they could not make these changes on their own.

SOCIAL FACTORS INFLUENCING DRINKING PATTERNS

For most people the peak drinking years are their late teens and early twenties. Thereafter consumption declines, particularly after retirement. Economic factors are probably very important in influencing consumption but changes in the individual's stage in their life-cycle and social role are also significant. A young working man or woman is relatively independent and has few commitments. On marriage, and particularly following the acquisition of a family, expectations and demands change and it is normally anticipated that less time will be spent outside the home drinking. Community studies of individuals who have moved out of problem drinking without the assistance of any formal agency suggest that factors such as marriage, a change of job, particularly where this is associated with reduced availability of alcohol, or a change in economic priorities, are important ingredients in precipitating change.

Family's responsibility in promoting sensible drinking

There is ample evidence that the attitude of the family is of great importance in influencing an individual's drinking. Most problems with alcohol are first recognized within the family. It is important that the family avoid covering up such a problem or colluding with the drinker by supporting denial and flimsy excuses. Those spouses who, within a supportive relationship, can confront each other with a realistic appraisal of the problems drinking is causing are most likely to achieve a successful resolution of the problem. Self-help measures often work best when family members take an active part in them.

Children are often surprised and even horrified as they grow up to find how like their parents they have become. At the age of eleven, Tom had often prayed that his father would stop drinking. He had seen him come home drunk and fight with his mother. He had sometimes found him lying on the kitchen floor and one night thought he was dead. He had always sworn that he would never drink and his mother had said that she hoped he would not grow up to be 'no good' like his father. Despite his early resolutions, Tom started drinking with friends at fifteen although he kept it a secret from his mother. However at sixteen, following a row with his mother, he went out and got very drunk. Looking back at the experience of his youth, he said: 'I suppose I had to show my mother then I was a man now and that I was independent.' His drinking quickly progressed to regular drunkenness. At the age of twenty-one, having been married for two years, he was in the habit of getting drunk and would often hit his wife when she criticized him. He suddenly realized that his pattern of behaviour had become almost identical to that which he had rejected in his father ten years earlier.

A familial trend in the acquisition of alcohol-related problems is well recognized (see Chapter 8). Part of this inheritance is genetic but the parent as role model for the child is a very important influence. Although a son or daughter may at first reject the way in which one or other parent misuses alcohol, they do none the less learn that alcohol is an important and powerful substance which can alleviate feelings or be used as a weapon in domestic arguments. Parents therefore should be conscious of the message they are conveying to their children by the way they drink and the importance they give to alcohol in everyday life.

Friendship and responsibility

Responsibility toward friends is also extremely important. In adolescence the peer group is a dominant influence in determining drinking patterns and such groups often reject or deprecate those who do not choose to drink alcohol. Every effort should be made to make it easier for young people to choose not to drink if that is their wish. Accepting differences between individuals is an aspect of maturity and the capacity to respect the choices of the other is an important attribute of friendship. Equally, friends need to be willing to allow their drinking companions to change their habits and not influence them into retaining a particular style by pressuring them to keep up with a drinking circle. Many problem drinkers find that pressure from friends is a common precipitant of relapse. Often this is because the friend who begins to curtail his or her own drinking makes the others uncomfortably conscious of their own habits.

Responsibility as host/hostess

A good host or hostess is often thought of as someone who makes sure that the guests have all they want to drink. They will ensure that no glass goes unfilled and that everyone drinks as much as they want. And yet, should good hosts provide their friends with the means of having a hangover, gastritis, or something worse, such as an accident? What is the responsibility of the dispenser for the consequences which follow? It is informative to contrast society's attitude toward the pusher of drugs and the dispenser of alcohol.

There have been a number of successful lawsuits in the United States brought against hosts and bar managers for allowing guests or customers to get into an inebriated state and thereby contribute to a subsequent accident. Without pursuing the philosophical and legal issues involved in the responsibility which one person has for another in these circumstances, there are a number of sensible guidelines which a good host might adopt for the welfare of his other guests.

1. Make sure that non-alcoholic drinks (including water) are readily and visibly available.

2. Try to ensure that food is also available when guests are drinking.

3. Never pressurize guests into drinking alcohol. Their refusal should always be accepted.

4. Do not top up glasses.

5. If someone seems to have drunk too much, don't offer them any more.

6. If there is any concern about a guest driving after drinking arrange a taxi or a lift home.

7. If you want to give someone a special alcoholic treat then emphasize quality rather than quantity.

Publicans should ensure that non-alcoholic drinks are clearly displayed and reasonably priced. There are of course laws governing the management of licensed premises which permit and even require publicans to refuse alcohol to someone who is evidently intoxicated. Such laws are very rarely enforced and could be much more widely employed.

Community

Many individuals feel powerless to exert any personal influence outside their family and friends. Beyond an occasional visit to the ballot box, they feel there is nothing which they personally can do about the overall level of drinking in their neighbourhood or community. This nihilism is not justified for there are a number of ways in which individuals or groups may have effective influence on the place of alcohol in their surroundings. These include taking an active interest in licensing changes and extensions of hours of opening, monitoring local drinks advertising, and forming local action groups around specific alcohol-related issues. For example, Mothers Against Drunk Driving (MADD) has proved an extremely influential pressure group in the United States and has had a definite impact on promoting greater concern about drinking and driving and road traffic safety. A similar pressure group the Campaign Against Drunk Driving (CADD) now exists in Britain. Professor Robinson and his colleagues at Hull

University have recently described in detail the ways in which local action may influence the level of alcohol misuse in a community.

Self-help groups

Alcoholics Anonymous was the prototype self-help group and its achievements have influenced many other special interest groups, such as Gamblers Anonymous and Narcotics Anonymous. The work of AA is described elsewhere (p. 160). The merits of self-help techniques have also led to the formation of groups such as Drinkwatchers concerned with monitoring personal alcohol consumption for non-alcohol dependent individuals who feel that their drinking is causing concern or becoming an excessive preoccupation.

CONCLUSION

A willingness to take a responsible attitude toward one's own drinking and a belief that it is possible for individuals to influence the behaviour and values of those around are essential components in curtailing the growth of alcohol problems.

10
What can be expected of treatment?

This chapter will not go into the technicalities of treatment methods for alcohol dependence and alcohol-related problems; such textbook considerations are outside the scope of this Report. However, to understand the role that treatment can play as a part of the country's total response to drinking problems, it is necessary to examine a number of issues. We need, for instance, to reconcile our emphasis on individual responsibility for drinking behaviour with the idea that such behaviour may indeed very much require outside assistance. How to overcome resistances to admitting the existence of a problem is again a question of more than technical importance. We shall examine some basic treatment assumptions, some of the usual treatment methods, and some of the current treatment controversies. Finally, we have to look at what treatment can be expected to achieve for the individual, and for society at large.

We should acknowledge from the outset that there are many influences in the pattern of services, not all of which have the problem drinkers' needs as their central concern. These include the nature of the area itself, i.e. whether it is urban or rural; the readiness of the community to give priority to developing services and the extent to which they can expect support from local and national politicians; the knowledge and skills of primary level health and social work staff; the importance accorded to cost effectiveness; the scarcity and geographical disposition of specialized teams, and the vision and enthusiasm of service planners and providers in public and voluntary services. These are a few examples of practical consideration which will shape services and give them a local flavour. None the less it seems reasonable to expect a basic minimum of provisions in any responsive and responsible community.

PATTERN OF TREATMENT

The evidence of earlier chapters makes it clear that the life of the problem drinker is replete with crises and at times disasters. He or she comes into conflict with family and friends; competence and reliability at work may suffer; accidents and illnesses recur and require treatment; law breaking and financial difficulties arise. This sad catalogue of incidents may be taken as evidence of the harm which alcohol may bring about; but it may also be taken as a listing of occasions and opportunities for intervention and change. The part which alcohol has played in bringing about the crisis may at first be concealed but the essence of help and treatment is to turn this crisis into an opportunity for change. The problem drinker's difficulties touch on a wide range of different agencies and individuals (see Figure 7).

Figure 7   *Levels of recognition and intervention*

level 1	the individual drinker (self-recognition)
	friends family
level 2	workmate social security
	barman
	employer police
level 3	social work General practitioner
	(primary health care team)
	hospital clergy marriage guidance council
level 4	alcohol problem services (NHS)
	Alcoholics Anonymous Council on Alcoholism

Note: See pp. 150–59 for explanation of levels. (At levels 2,3,4 examples only are given and the lists are not intended to be exhaustive.)

At the first level is the drinker who may recognize the nature of the problem and either finds that he or she can cut back to less damaging drinking using self-help techniques described in Chapter 9 or else decide to seek further outside assistance. Family and friends are also placed at this first level because they play a key role in confronting the drinker with the problem and in facilitating recovery.

At the next level is an array of individuals who certainly can recognize that a problem exists and may be well placed to give advice and initiate referral. For example, the success and benefits of alcohol in employment policies (p. 164) rests on the willingness of workmates, and particularly supervisors, to recognize and refer colleagues whose work is deteriorating. In some countries bar tenders have been trained to recognize and advise clients whose drinking is clearly causing them problems.

At the next level is an array of primary health and social work agencies. They do not have alcohol problems as a priority concern but the consequences of alcohol misuse contribute greatly to their case loads. They are very well placed to recognize and deal with alcohol problems, often at an early stage before serious consequences and losses have occurred. A great deal of current treatment philosophy is devoted to enhancing skills at this level, particularly for social workers and members of the primary health care teams (see pp. 168–69).

Finally, there are specialist resources provided either by health and social workers or by voluntary agencies. They provide specialist consultative training and support to the other levels as well as offering direct services usually for the more complex and advanced forms of alcohol problems.

THE PROCESS OF CHANGING HABITS

As discussed in Chapter 9, some people with drinking problems are able to deal with their own behaviour without recourse to professional or organized help, and there is good evidence that this is happening in the community all the time. A drinking problem should be a signal for self-questioning and sensible change. Here is an example of a story that is not uncommon:

> 'When I was in the forces and the war had ended and we were all hanging about with nothing to do, I drank like a fish. Makes me shudder to think about it now – the risks we took driving back to the camp at night. My fiancée broke off our engagement, and I couldn't blame her. When I came back to civvy street, I got in straightaway with a lot of drinkers, and went on knocking the stuff back. I suppose I was about through with spending my gratuity, a lot of money gone, when I said to myself, "This has got to stop". And it meant finding entirely different friends, taking up new leisure interests, and chucking in the rugger club, and more than anything making up my mind as to what I actually meant to do with my life,

rather than just drifting along in a boozy haze. I met another girl I very much liked, and I certainly wasn't going to ruin things again.'

Not everyone's self-determination may have to be harnessed to so serious a problem as that described by the man quoted above, but the practical message is that many people will at some time in their lives have to make small or large modifications in their drinking behaviour, and that the capacity for making such changes often lies well within their powers. They will be much aided by the understanding (and demands) of their families and others around them. (The problem is contained and catered for within level one of Figure 7.)

If the simple view were accepted that a drinking problem automatically necessitated professional treatment, then there would be no confusion. But a dilemma inevitably results when it is accepted that some people may be able to do all that is needed by means of their own resources (with society encouraging this view of self-determination), while the message is at the same time given that other people should indeed seek professional help (and should be encouraged to do so without delays which can result in unnecessary further harm). A balance must obviously be struck, and it is not absolutely different in kind from the decisions that people make every day on a host of other medical and social issues – whether for instance a headache is a pain to be endured, dealt with by going to bed early or by taking a pain killer, or a symptom which requires a visit to the doctor.

We do not wish to discourage appropriate help-seeking, but to encourage everyone's sense of personal responsibility. Some people who are drinking harmfully, and certainly those who have become severely dependent, may well find it impossible to deal with their situations without some degree of special help. The present lack of information on the nature of dependence means that someone may not even have a clear idea of what he or she has to deal with, until some informed advice can be obtained.

ACKNOWLEDGING THE PROBLEM

The common starting point for any constructive changes in behaviour is often the individual's personal realization and admission that drinking is causing a problem; this is equally true whether an individual is going to remedy the matter by his or her own efforts, or with professional help, or by joining Alcoholics Anonymous. Unfortunately, it is commonly believed that the 'typical' drinker with a desperately severe problem will adamantly refuse to admit that a problem exists at all, and will stubbornly refuse help despite the manifest damage that is being caused to themselves and their friends and family. Such sad instances occur on occasion, but it is wrong to take the extreme case as typical. In every case, facing up to the facts will be an important personal issue, but it is a matter of degree, and we should not assume that extreme denial is always involved, or that it will last for ever.

Of course, the problem of facing worrying facts is not unique to drinking. If someone is frightened or ashamed of their behaviour, they are likely to hide or deny what they are doing; this is an understandable defensive strategy. If the drinker is then simply scolded in an unconstructive fashion, the denial is likely to become more determined. Excessive drinking may often lead to behaviour that is worrying or shaming for the person concerned, and some degree of resistance to seeing the true facts of the situation is therefore hardly surprising.

The problem drinker is ambivalent about making changes and uses various psychological strategies or defences against acknowledging the disturbing fact that alcohol has caused problems. The individual is aware of the desire to continue drinking and the desire to stop taking alcohol or at least to control its use. This conflict is uncomfortable, as with other conflicts, and to resolve it the individual has essentially two alternatives. These are to modify the drinking to the desired goal, or to leave the drinking as it is but to use psychological defence mechanisms to prevent the reality of the situation being made clear. These include projection (i.e. blaming others), or the rationalization that the drinking is not causing any harm, or passivity whereby the individual considers it is impossible to change. This conflict around accepting undesirable facts is an extremely important part of the way the individual deals with an alcohol problem and it must be clearly recognized by the therapist. The drinker's decision hangs in the balance and many individuals will not modify their drinking behaviour unless they clearly see that the harm from continued drinking outweighs the rewards. This conflict is a dynamic one and can change from minute to minute as well as from day to day, as resolution waxes and wanes. In our culture the conflict is frequently more intense for women who often feel a greater degree of shame about their drinking and find it difficult to acknowledge the extent of their drinking to others.

There are several ways to deal with resistance of this sort, and overcoming resistance is more often a matter of whittling it away than dealing with it at a stroke.

'Well, I knew he'd got a drinking problem, but for some time he just wouldn't take any notice of what I said. He'd try to avoid the issue, or fly into a rage and put all the blame on me. It went on for a couple of years that way. He wouldn't go to the doctor. I tried leaving AA pamphlets around but he took no more notice of them than of all the bills he didn't pay. I think what finally got through to him was when his brother had a word, and he could see that we were all on his side.'

In addition to the pressures from family or friends, the general climate of attitudes and stock of ideas that society provides with regard to drinking behaviour will also be important, together with more general social attitudes towards deviance, towards the ability to admit problems or to seek help, and so on. If society could more readily accept the idea that drinking problems are common and do not have to be shamefully hidden, then it might indeed be easier for the troubled person to surrender denial earlier.

If a person with a drinking problem feels under severe and unsympathetic attack, further barriers may be put up; but if people just say nothing or join in the conspiracy of denial, something even less helpful is done. Both the initiation of change in drinking behaviour and the continued support of the individual who is trying to alter a harmful drinking pattern must therefore be seen as usually dependent on interactions with family and friends, rather than lying only with the individual, or only with the professionals. Workmates and others who encounter the problem drinker in his or her daily activities can help by being tactfully open about the problems they observe and offering advice about sources of help where possible (level 2 in Figure 7).

Readiness to make use of professional help (or to turn to Alcoholics Anonymous) must then depend not only on actual willingness to admit a problem, but also on factual knowledge about where help may be found, readiness of access, and the attitudes of the professionals when approached. Resistance to recognizing drinking problems or unwillingness to take a constructive and helpful attitude may, on occasion, reside with the professionals as much as with the drinker. The resistances and denials of the doctor who 'never sees drinking problems in his practice' are targets for education.

SOME BASIC TREATMENT ASSUMPTIONS

This section describes some basic ideas which underlie the treatment of alcohol-related problems. The aim is to provide a general understanding of the treatment that can be provided at the primary level of care (level 3 in Figure 7).

The drinking problem: to be taken seriously but never as the exclusive focus

Anyone who has had experience with the treatment of alcohol dependence will realize that the drinking problem does not exist in isolation. Likewise, patients sometimes complain that 'drink isn't really the problem'. Such objections rightly remind us that it is a person who is coming for help, with an essential sense of being a person with various troubles and perplexities which exist in their own right, and which may predate the excessive drinking, or cause it, or intertwine with it, or exacerbate it. The balance always has to be struck between an insistent awareness of the importance of drinking in the total picture, and the fact that excessive drinking is highly unlikely to be the only problem experienced by the client. The helping agent who is going to respond to the client, besides having knowledge of drinking problems, has to be capable therefore of a wide perspective: the person required is the general practitioner, the social worker with general training, the psychiatrist or physician with a good general knowledge of his subject, and so on. The philosophy and techniques of Alcoholics Anonymous show in well-developed form this ability to respond to drinking in proper perspective: AA is about coming to terms with alcoholism, but also about coming to terms with oneself, with one's relationships, and with surrounding realities. The basic skill at this stage is an ability to help the alcohol-dependent person make a clear link between alcohol and the problems which beset him or her.

The need for a thorough case assessment

Where there is a drinking problem of any complexity, a two-minute interview is not going to provide the necessary basis of understanding on which to formulate a treatment approach that is personal to the needs of that particular sufferer and his or her family. A full assessment must be social, as well as medical and psychological, and may have to involve interviews with the family as well as with the client.

Gathering a full case history may be important not only for the information that it gives the doctor or social worker or the treatment team, but also in terms of its unique significance for that individual. The business of sharing in a review of the present situation and its historical development, the sympathetic invitation to openness, and the conduct of a kind of self-audit, can provide a new self-awareness on which much else can subsequently be built.

Identifying goals

In helping the drinker achieve changes there are special reasons for an emphasis on identifying therapeutic goals (which must again be specific to the particular person and family). Clear goals help to relieve the sense of chaos, of 'everything piling in upon me', and make movement towards recovery possible. Goals may, for instance, relate to physical or psychological health, to the functioning of the marriage, or to social matters such as getting a new job or moving to a better home. Obviously, one important goal must relate to the drinking behaviour – and here the goal may be abstinence (as is usually the case where the person is severely dependent upon alcohol), or the modification of drinking towards a more acceptable pattern. A set of multiple goals has to be developed, rather than a drinking goal only. Goals have to be step-wise and realistic, rather than so ambitiously set from the start as to be defeating. They cannot be imposed, but have to be negotiated with the client and the family.

The essence of effective treatment often lies in the skill shown in handling such a matter as the setting of goals. A visible target as to what is to be achieved – 'I will take my son to football matches on Saturday afternoons' – restores to the troubled individual some small immediate sense of his own powers and possibilities.

From such small but significant beginnings the drinker can build towards major changes in style of life, finding rewarding alternatives to the time spent drinking, and developing a new set of personal values. Such major reconstruction work takes time and will probably involve setbacks. The important ingredients which the therapist can offer at an early stage are hope and confidence that the changes can be achieved.

Working towards agreed objectives

We have discussed the importance of the client's self-responsibility, and emphasized that any intervention should seek to maximize rather than undermine that individual's sense of responsibility. Treatment must also support, and find alliance with, the helping resources of family and community. Professional guidance may be needed on how best to find the way of achieving the desired goals; this help may be in the form of relatively brief counselling, or longer-term assistance. On occasion it may be clear that intensive or specialized help is needed if the client is to be enabled to learn self-help; initially admission to hospital may be necessary to prevent, or to receive treatment for, severe withdrawal symptoms; physical health may have to be restored; an underlying depressive illness may have to be treated; or a 'Skid Row' alcoholic may have to be found a hostel place and given a way out of a circular and destructive process of degradation.

Goals are thus reached by a variety of methods and often by a variety of forms of co-operation; the sufferer's own commitment and involvement are essential, the family and the immediate social environment often have an important part to play, while professional help, counsellors, and Alcoholics Anonymous can provide ancillary assistance if they are deployed sensitively and with due regard to the whole person and the family.

Continuing care and relapse management

Another treatment principle, which is gaining general acceptance, is that patients with the more severe type of drinking problem should be offered continuing contact with a helping agency, at least for the first year or two after commencing treatment. Drinking problems of any severity are never resolved overnight; a patient's greater awareness of problems often evolves slowly and the wish for help may similarly evolve. Relapse is inevitably quite a frequent occurrence so that further crisis help may be needed along the way. Some sort of continued availability on the part of the helper, and an assurance to the patient that someone will continue to be interested, is therefore often indicated. A regular reminder that the venture is worthwhile and the repeated instillation of hope at times of despair and crisis are both invaluable ingredients of effective therapy.

Relapses will most often occur within the first few months of therapy. Neither the problem drinker nor the family should regard these as catastrophic provided they are attended to promptly and continued contact with the treatment agency is maintained. They should, however, be taken seriously and viewed as an opportunity for enhanced self-understanding and appreciation of the precipitants involved. Many relapses occur in response to deeply felt emotions and anxieties or interpersonal stress, or from an inability to withstand environmental pressures to drink. Patients who have carefully rehearsed a repertoire of techniques for coping with these pressures have a better chance of avoiding relapse. It also helps if the likely consequences of relapse can be vividly retained in the patient's mind as this seems to offset the understandable temptation to think only of the short-term spurious benefits which might follow a return to former habits.

For example, Charlotte recognized that relapses commonly occurred on Thursday nights before the children, who were at boarding school, came home for the weekend. She would work vigorously in the house during the week so that it would be tidy and 'perfect' for their return so they could enjoy the weekend. She would then get so drunk on Thursday and Friday that she would be incapable of meeting them. They would have to look after her and the weekend would be 'ruined'.

She planned ways of avoiding this critical series of events. She would arrange to visit a friend who knew of her drinking problem on Thursday evening. On Fridays she would go walking with the dogs and spend a lot of time having a leisurely bath and relaxing listening to her favourite music. These activities were both rewarding and helped her handle the mounting anxiety she often felt during that time. If the anxiety became worse she was encouraged to phone a friend or counsellor and talk about how she was feeling. Along with these measures she also retained a vivid mental imagery of herself lying on the sofa when the children came home, unable to get up, her dress stained with vomit. These were, of course, short-term psychological devices that helped her to cope in the first few months of abstinence while she effected more lasting changes in her way of life.

Detoxification

Alcohol withdrawal symptoms have been described in a previous chapter (pp. 58–9, 63); they range from the trivial to the markedly unpleasant and life threatening (delirium tremens or withdrawal fits). A patient suffering from the dependence syndrome may, therefore, require immediate specialized medical assistance in 'coming off' alcohol. This may be accomplished with a GP's help or on an out-patient basis if social support is available, but severe dependence is sometimes an indication for hospital admission so that careful observation can be provided, and intensive nursing and medical care are on hand. A variety of drugs may be used to provide pharmacological cover for withdrawal, and specially skilled nursing may be needed for the delirious and agitated patient. Modern methods of care are very successful in treating this acute phase of the problem, and risks to life have been much reduced. The development of detoxification centres over the last few years has shown that alcohol dependents, including those on 'Skid Row', can be safely and effectively treated in such centres and they provide an important alternative to the use of the police cell as a detoxification centre. Detoxification can usually be achieved in a non-medical setting provided medical services are readily available when necessary. Regrettably, there is now little, if any, government support for any long-term plans for detoxification centres.

⌈SPECIAL TREATMENT METHODS IN OUTLINE⌉

In the preceding section some general principles of treatment have been discussed. Such processes as making the assessment, agreeing on goals, and discussing how goals are to be reached, may be extremely important therapeutic influences in their own right. But special techniques may have a part to play, employed within the context of these more general influences. The paragraphs below are not to be taken as listing techniques in order of usefulness: the possible value of any technique must depend on the individual patient – they are principally but not exclusively provided by the more specialist resources (level 4 in Figure 7).

Psychotherapy

The principal therapeutic tool used in many alcohol problem clinics and therapeutic hostels, and indeed in a form in Alcoholics Anonymous, is the group therapy approach. Such group therapies have the common features of identification, confession, emotional arousal, implantation of new ideas, and long-term support by fellow members of the group. Individual psychotherapy may also have a place, though this is not as favoured as therapy in the group setting. Clearly, family therapy or marital therapy involving both client and spouse or 'both partners' may also be important. Sexual difficulties are not likely to improve, using sexual therapy techniques, unless an individual has been abstinent for some period.

Marital and family therapy

The importance of the family in both the genesis of and recovery from alcohol problems has been stressed throughout this book. Many therapists now regard the participation of the patient's spouse and sometimes other family members as an essential ingredient of recovery. The spouse of the problem drinker often needs an opportunity to discuss the stresses which the family has experienced and to obtain information about the nature of drinking problems. Some therapists have endeavoured to move away from a patient-centred approach to alcohol problems and have come to regard the drinking as one facet of a disturbed family system. In consequence they focus attention on this system itself. Whichever theoretical approach is adopted it is clear that the family will have to undergo significant readjustments as the problem drinker finds a new style of life. There is good evidence that a spouse who is supportive but does not collude with the drinker's evasions or minimize the seriousness of the drinking problem, makes a major contribution to a favourable treatment outcome.

Women's groups

As increasing numbers of women develop alcohol-related problems it has become evident that programmes must accommodate to their specific needs. Women commonly feel more guilty and stigmatized about having a drinking problem and some may find it easier to speak freely if they can have part of their treatment within a service for women only. In such a setting they find it easier to talk openly about their difficulties and particularly to discuss some of the sexual abuses many women alcoholics have experienced. In facilitating access to treatment for women additional services such as neighbourhood based clinics and the provision of creches are important considerations.

Alcoholics Anonymous, Al-Anon, and Al-Ateen

Alcoholics Anonymous celebrated its fiftieth anniversary in 1985 and claims worldwide to have helped more than a million members. It is unwise for anyone who is significantly alcohol dependent not to have at least looked very closely at AA. This is often best achieved through initial personal introduction to a member of AA with whom the problem drinker can identify. It is too much to expect the drinker just to go to a meeting. It usually requires fifteen to twenty meetings at more than one group before any sensible opinion can be made about its value for an individual. Many people have found in AA exactly the help and understanding they require, others may take something from AA's philosophy, but not become regular attenders. Al-Anon, an organization for relatives and friends of alcoholics, deserves similar recognition as an extremely valuable resource. It is well worth exploring by anyone closely involved with a problem drinker, as it teaches the relative how best to deal with the difficulties of living with an alcoholic. A relative or friend may join Al-Anon and find support there even when the drinking partner is unwilling to recognize or deal with the problem. Al-Ateen has evolved specially for the teenage children of alcoholics.

Alcoholics Anonymous provides a fellowship which encourages frankness about alcohol problems in a group surrounded by others who can readily identify with the drinker's suffering and shame and at the same time offers support in finding a new way of life. AA firmly believes that abstinence is the only route to recovery for those who regard themselves as 'truly alcoholic'. Drinkwatchers is another self-help organization which is concerned to help those who are consuming alcohol in a hazardous way to return to less damaging drinking habits.

Behaviour therapies

Behaviour therapies, in contrast to more analytic and insight orientated therapies, aim to treat the 'problem behaviour' directly, rather than via

What can be expected of treatment?

the supposed underlying psychodynamic or personality probl[em].
Aversion therapies in which clients learned to associate drinking [with]
pain or vomiting have largely fallen into disuse. Most modern
behaviour therapies are based on the belief that what is required is the
learning of new behaviours while discarding old ones. It includes
simply teaching a patient to be able to say 'no' when offered a drink,
teaching alternative skills such as relaxation with which to meet stress
or tension rather than resorting to drink, teaching the person to drink
more moderately and to judge personal blood-alcohol level, or
teaching how to put up with slight withdrawal symptoms without taking
a morning drink and becoming involved again in a cycle of drinking.
Learning social skills, particularly assertiveness, is often a benefit to
those who drink in order to overcome shyness or feel unable to cope
with certain social situations. Some psychologists today favour the use
of a combination of several behaviour techniques tailored to the
individual patient's needs – a 'broad spectrum' approach.

Deterrent drugs

Disulfiram (Antabuse) was introduced into clinical practice in 1948.
The individual who takes the tablets regularly and who then drinks will
become nauseated, flushed, and generally feel ill. Disulfiram thus
serves as a sort of chemical fence around their drinking. Nowadays, it
is becoming more frequent for the doctor to suggest that a third person
supervise the Antabuse, for example, a clinic staff nurse or other
helper, a relative, or someone at work. Shock or rarely death can result
if a patient drinks heavily when he is taking a full dose of tablets, so this
is not a treatment that can be given without explanation, a prior
medical assessment, and continuing medical supervision. It is not
suitable for every problem drinker and should not be undertaken
without serious commitment. The drug fell into disrepute because
some patients found that if taking it irregularly they could after forty-
eight hours drink with impunity although for others the effects were
evident for a week or more. Supervision by a third person imposes a
valuable extra control, because as long as the subject is taking the drug
he is unable to drink and, knowing that he cannot, often feels much
less craving. While abstinence is assured, the patient can begin to
readjust to a different life, find new ways of coping with problems and,
in time, rebuild relationships with family, friends, and work colleagues.
Patients should continue to receive help in these areas and not regard
the pill as a panacea, otherwise relapse commonly occurs as soon as the
patient stops taking the drug. There is no medical limit on how long
Antabuse can be taken. Most individuals who use the tablets

successfully for six or twelve months feel they would like to try to do without them but others prefer to continue taking them for years on end.

In-patient admission

There is no doubt that some of those who suffer from alcohol problems will require in-patient care although it is quite wrong to see this as a panacea or optimum solution to a drinking problem. Admission may be indicated for a variety of physical and psychological complications. These include the immediate protection of the individual's life, sometimes for the relief of the acutely threatening impact of his behaviour on others or, on occasions, for detoxification. In other circumstances admission will be required for detailed assessment or intensive psychotherapy for underlying psychological problems. Whether in-patient care is indicated simply for the treatment of the drinking habit itself (by means, for instance, of group psychotherapy) is to be decided only with reference to the particular patient. A recent survey of alcoholism treatment units found that the majority had as part of their programme a course of in-patient psychotherapy. In many circumstances day patient treatment alone will prove sufficient.

SOME TREATMENT CONTROVERSIES

Thus far we have attempted a broad sketch of what treatment is about in terms that might generally be accepted by most professionals who practise in this field. Some note must now be taken of issues on which there would at present be greater diversity of opinion. Anyone studying the medical, social, and psychological approaches available is immediately struck by their diversity; it is a time when many methods are being tried, partly in recognition of the diverse forms of alcohol problems.

Optimum pattern of services

There is continuing debate about the optimum balance of specialist as opposed to generalist primary level services. The creation of a cadre of specialists of sufficient size to respond directly to most alcohol-related problems is clearly uneconomic and undesirable. The trend has therefore been toward ensuring that the care-givers who make first contact have the skills and knowledge to enable them to recognize and respond effectively to problem drinkers and their families. In some cases this intervention will be sufficient but others will require specialist support or consultation. Specialist services are therefore likely to devote their scarce resources to helping the more complex and intractable cases and providing support, consultation, information, and education to primary level agencies. Such a strategy implies a local support network of adequately trained specialists.

The Royal College of Psychiatrists has suggested that each region should have a consultant psychiatrist who has received specialist training in alcohol and drug misuse problems. In a few regions there have also been plans to appoint a consultant physician with a similar special interest.

A further development has been the creation of Community Alcohol Teams. These are groups of professionals who will assist primary care agents in dealing with problem drinkers and alcohol dependent individuals and also help in providing consultation to a network of services. The recent expansion of the Councils on Alcoholism with trained and other non-statutory services such as Accept and Industrial Alcoholism Units or employee assistance programmes have provided a valuable new resource, both relieving the specialist services and being a point at which the individual or his concerned family or employer can make a direct contact. These specialist resources are all heavily reliant on the skills of the primary level agencies such as general practitioners, social workers, and in some areas police who will be the first point of contact for most problem drinkers.

General practitioner

General practitioners are well placed to detect people who are abusing alcohol and who are either at risk of developing problems or have already done so. Few problem drinkers will seek help or advice from agencies of any type about their drink problems, particularly while these are at an early stage. However, the great majority of such drinkers, in common with the rest of the population, will see their GP at least once a year, even if the consultation is not directly related to their problem drinking.

Thus the general practitioner is in an ideal position to intervene in early problem drinking, once the patients can be identified. Unfortunately many general practitioners feel pessimistic about being able to help problem drinkers, a view which would need to change before effective help is possible. Over the past decade, a number of biochemical tests have been developed and refined which constitute useful markers of chronic excessive alcohol consumption. In addition, a number of simple, easy-to-administer, and brief questionnaires have been devised to help in detection and the combination of biochemical tests and questionnaires have helped doctors and others to identify problem drinkers with greater ease.

Clinical practice suggests that GP intervention, though brief and simple, can be very effective. While it has not been established, the hope is that many people who are drinking heavily might be persuaded to modify their drinking *before* proceeding to develop serious physical, psychological, and/or social problems. The provision of factual information concerning drink and its impact, with advice tailored to the individual patient, coupled with follow-up assessments on a regular basis to monitor response, are important tasks for the GP.

Employee assistance programmes

Alcohol problems frequently manifest as impaired work performance. This fact can be turned to therapeutic advantage by the creation of 'employee assistance programmes' whereby a company establishes a policy for dealing with employees whose work performance is impaired by alcohol misuse or other factors. The policy needs to be developed in joint consultation between union and management and applied equally to *all* levels within the organization, i.e. in the boardroom as well as on the shop floor. If alcohol appears to be affecting an employee's work performance then he or she can choose to accept referral to an appropriate source of help with guaranteed continued employment provided they co-operate with treatment. The employee may of course reject such a course of action and accept ordinary disciplinary procedures, but in companies where such policies exist and are genuinely operated the extra motivation provided by the opportunity to remain employed greatly enhanced treatment outcome.

Return to normal drinking

A further recent development and a matter for lively debate is the drinking goal to be recommended for the particular patient – a question which has already been touched on (p. 156). Until recently, lifelong abstinence would have been the only goal that could be offered responsibly to a patient who showed evidence of the dependence syndrome. This view has been challenged by those who consider it to be too absolute, and who have produced careful research to show that a small number of patients who have developed dependence may later regain a seemingly confident control over their drinking. The controversy has sometimes been fierce, and still continues. It is best to admit that the 'return to normal drinking' argument is at present not fully resolved, and to acknowledge that an individual judgement is needed in each case, made after discussing with the drinker both what is desirable and what is feasible.

ALCOHOL AND OTHER FORMS OF DRUG ABUSE

Many alcohol abusers also misuse prescribed and illicit drugs. Other forms of substance abuse are the subject of a forthcoming report by this College and will not be discussed here. None the less there is considerable debate at present concerning the wisdom of combining treatment resources for alcohol dependents with facilities for those who are addicted to other drugs. To some extent the services must overlap because the different forms of misuse coexist with the same individual. For instance, the treatment of alcohol withdrawal is commonly complicated by dependence on tranquillizers such as Librium or Valium. There are also similarities between the processes of becoming dependent on alcohol and other drugs – they can often be studied and understood within identical scientific frames of reference. In many respects it makes sense to plan jointly for all forms of substance misuse while acknowledging and catering for the unique aspects of each form of dependence.

Type of treatment

Additional controversies exist as to which type of special technique is appropriate in what circumstances – whether psychotherapy or behaviour therapy is to be employed, the drug of choice for withdrawal, whether family therapy is indicated, and so on. There can be no doubt that the whole area of treatment stands much in need of research which can provide objective answers to these many questions, large and small.

WHAT CAN BE EXPECTED OF TREATMENT?

Treatment for alcohol dependence

So much for a general account of what is meant by treatment, and of the current debates. In the light of what has been said here, what place should be accorded to treatment services within the total strategy of the country's response to drinking problems? Evidence as to the actual efficacy of treatment is in some ways still surprisingly scant. The published research deals almost exclusively with treatment of patients suffering from problems of such degree as to qualify for referral to psychiatric hospitals, where the diagnosis of 'alcoholism' is often the starting point for selection and entry to treatment. It may be presumed that such patients are likely to have been severely dependent. In the past abstinence has nearly always been the goal which has been advised and against which efficacy has been gauged.

Reports from Britain and other countries concur in suggesting that about 60 per cent of patients of this type who attend clinics will show worthwhile or substantial improvement at the end of a twelve-month follow-up, although less than half of that 60 per cent will have achieved complete or nearly complete abstinence for the full twelve months. Multiple measures of change will often be employed, including not only changes in drinking behaviour, but work status, criminal behaviour, marital adjustment, physical health, and various psychological measures. Drinking less is usually, but not always, related to improvement in these other measures. Outcome after one year is generally thought to be a fair pointer to subsequent prognosis, although some patients will certainly relapse later on, either transiently or more disastrously. Others may begin to show significant improvement only after a longer struggle.

However, there are some caveats to the full significance to be accorded the sort of figures just quoted. First, it has to be noted that about 40 per cent of patients appear to derive little benefit from the best endeavours of the treatment services, at least over the usual period of observation. With such a potentially devastating condition as alcoholism a 60 per cent success rate is cause for optimism, but the fact that treatment fails to benefit another significant proportion of patients cannot be left out of the reckoning. It must also be noted that the sort of success rate that we are quoting here is the type of result that is generally reported from specialized units which have a fairly rigorous process of patient selection. Indeed, even more rigorous screening, accepting for treatment only patients with the most favourable outlook, will result in a success rate considerably above the one that we have given. Even levels of around 60 per cent success are, however, usually based on selection of patients who are to a considerable extent 'motivated for treatment', and it is not unusual for patients with 'severe personality disorder' to be rejected at the initial screening, for patients with severe physical damage (and particularly brain damage) to be selected out as 'too deteriorated', while homeless alcoholics are also often excluded. The overall impact of the selection process may therefore produce, as the basis for the research report, a group of patients with a personality profile and degree of social stability which are atypical of the larger reality of all those who come to hospitals for help. Good results can to an extent be obtained by stacking the cards in this way, and results from centres where case selection has been less rigorous do not look so promising – a favourable outcome may then be obtained with only 20 to 30 per cent of subjects and it becomes hard to demonstrate that treatment itself is having any lasting benefit. Instead it may only be providing first aid and tiding people over crises. First aid and bringing comfort are, of course, part of a long established medical and caring tradition which is of short-term humanitarian value in itself. This is not to suggest that the results obtained from specialized treatment services should be considered in any way spurious, or that they should be discounted. They speak, however, only of the type of result which can be expected with a segment of the total case load.

Scientific evaluation of the effectiveness of treatment is extremely difficult but its complexity must not be brushed aside in our eagerness to know if a new approach 'works'. If evaluation is fudged then the true effectiveness of different therapies will never be known. Different approaches need to be offered to groups of patients who are comparable in terms of social stability, degree of dependence, and so on. Outcome needs to be contrasted with the spontaneous changes which occur in drinking patterns even among dependent drinkers. Compliance with the treatment offered also needs taking into account. Far fewer people with alcohol problems comply with treatment than patients with medical and psychiatric disorders. It is difficult to form an opinion about a specific treatment for problem drinkers when it is abandoned prematurely by at least half. Improving compliance with and commitment to treatment is a major challenge to the future development of services.

Still focusing only on the patient with the dependence syndrome or with the more serious type of drinking problem, we then have to consider the question of what percentage of all such persons in the community are, in practice, making contact with helping agencies. The ideal way to answer this question would be to conduct a survey which would identify and enumerate all individuals in a given community with serious drinking problems, and then determine what proportion of these were in contact with helping agencies. Such research is difficult and expensive, and has seldom been attempted, but a limited project bearing on this question was conducted in Camberwell in 1966. It revealed that only 11 to 22 per cent of people with a serious drinking problem had been in contact with an appropriate agency during the previous year.

Taking another set of figures, DHSS data suggest that there are currently about 14,500 admissions annually to NHS hospitals in

England and Wales for treatment of alcoholism; this has to be set against estimates of the total national prevalence of alcoholism which range between 300,000 and 500,000. The contribution of non-specialist agencies, particularly the general practitioner, out-patient care, private practice, voluntary agencies, and Alcoholics Anonymous, would have to be added to these DHSS in-patient admission figures. These additional numbers may be considerable – for example, Scotland's Council on Alcoholism see about 6,000 clients a year. But by any reckoning it does appear that the treatment system (even defined in the broadest sense), is at present reaching only a rather small proportion of those who stand in need.

One response to this type of calculation, which sets out the probable ratio between the size of the problem population and the extent of treatment actually delivered, would be to argue that the figures clearly show the need to increase the treatment facilities and to run a more active campaign to bring people into treatment. Such a policy might be expected to bring benefits, but it also seems possible that a law of diminishing returns might begin to operate: there may be a limit to the proportion of those with serious drinking problems who are willing to enrol as 'patients' or are able to benefit from the available treatments. There will also be a limit to the country's willingness and capacity to allocate resources to the costs of providing services to problem drinkers, since it is only one among the many demands on the budget and human resources of the NHS. Treatment certainly has a vital, continuing, and evolving place within the total strategy of the country's response to alcohol-related problems, but the facts suggest that it would be misleading to hope that specialist services could be so developed that the majority of people with serious drinking problems could ever be brought into treatment and effectively treated.

So far the discussion has centred on the type of person who is sufficiently badly affected by his drinking to become a patient in a psychiatric hospital or special alcoholism unit, or to figure in the DHSS 'alcoholism' statistics, or to be identified in a community survey as having a serious drinking problem.

Early intervention

One avenue of hope, recently supported by research, is that of identifying problem drinkers at a stage before they are severely dependent or have inevitably damaged their social network and employment prospects. It has been demonstrated that in these early cases clear unequivocal advice given in a non-judgemental manner, which helps the excessive drinker weigh up the advantages and disadvantages of his life style, has a discernible benefit, possibly over several years if the brief contact is repeated. So far this has been shown in general hospitals and medical screening centres, but the efficacy of the approach in general practice is also being studied.

Can treatment be the major national strategy?

Such early intervention could in theory be extended to those who have contact with the social work, police or other statutory services, and though we have no evidence as yet that it would be effective, research might eventually reveal a subsection who would respond. Most harmful effects of drinking are not accounted for by that relatively small number of severely dependent people to whom the treatment services are directed, but by moderate and heavy drinkers, as stated on p. 110. There has to be a sense of perspective. Treatment will, for instance, help some drunken drivers and there is an urgent need for research such as that started by the Department of Transport into identifying those with serious drinking problems who would benefit from treatment. But surely we cannot hope to meet the drunk driving problem, or many other similar problems, with a cry for 'more treatment', although early intervention policies might be expected to improve matters.

In summary, we believe that two equally essential conclusions should be drawn as to what society may expect of treatment. The first conclusion is that treatment very often has something vitally important to offer: the person who is worried about his or her drinking should know that if they cannot deal with things alone it is definitely in their interests to seek professional advice, go to Alcoholics Anonymous or a local council on alcoholism, and to do so early. Treatment services need to be strengthened to allow this. But the second conclusion (which in no way contradicts the first) is that, in terms of national strategies, the contribution that treatment can be expected to make is definitely limited. In the final chapter we shall consider how these appraisals bear on recommendations for future national strategies, both for treatment and for the prevention of drinking problems.

11
A better response in the future

Lives are being ruined on a large scale by the misuse of alcohol. It is easy to become so dulled by the toll of casualties that we do not notice the magnitude of the suffering. We cease to look behind the statistics, and forget that each death from cirrhosis represents the end of a very personal tragedy, and that the human wreck dozing with a meths bottle on the park bench is someone's son or daughter, husband or wife, or that the young person severely injured in a drunk driving accident is left with a lifetime of pain, disability, and regret. We ignore these visible manifestations of society's inability to cope with the alcohol problem only at our long-term peril. In most industrialized and developing countries alcohol consumption has risen steadily since the Second World War, and alcohol-related disabilities are on the increase in most parts of the world. We may try to comfort ourselves with the knowledge that there are countries with more serious problems than Britain, but the sort of data that this Report has presented on our own national scale should quickly dispel any sense of self-satisfaction.

The key facts have been stated in earlier chapters. They make it plain that although there has been some recent levelling off in per capita consumption and in the prevalence of some alcohol problems, the cost to the community remains much too high for us to tolerate. Recollect that for alcohol misuse the economic cost alone was conservatively estimated to be £1,614 million in 1983.

In this chapter a number of recommendations will be made. Some remain unchanged from the first report of this College because they are just as salient as they were seven years ago, others point to new directions for future developments. These suggestions will deal as much with ways of looking at problems as with practical actions: the two aspects are equally vital. To make recommendations is of course to risk being attacked for being too vague, too assured, or plain wrong-headed. These risks are taken in the belief that a report of this nature must reach conclusions rather than dodge every issue as being too difficult, insufficiently researched, or somebody else's business: the crucial issues with alcohol problems are too often evaded. Denial is not the sole prerogative of the sufferer. It is not, however, presumed that these recommendations constitute some sort of grand or grandiose blueprint: they are offered as a starting point.

PREVENTION

The need for an emphasis on prevention

We believe that prevention is still receiving pitifully inadequate attention although funding has improved somewhat since the time of the College's first report. In this regard alcohol problems are no exception to the general pattern of preventive health expenditure in this country, and indeed most other parts of the world. Gigantic and increasing sums are being spent on the treatment of illness, while the prevention of ill health is a notion more honoured in principle than in practice. About £13,000 million is now spent annually in Britain on the National Health Service, and of this huge sum less than 6 per cent is devoted to preventive work. In 1984 the total spent on advertising by the beer industry alone was nearly £80 million. The total budget allocated to the Health Education Council for the whole range of its activities on every health topic was £9 million.

We make the recommendation that:

● **Health policies on alcohol problems should give much greater attention to prevention than has previously been the case.**

Our recommendations on prevention are in line with views expressed in the report of the Expenditure Committee of the House of Commons, and also with those of the Report on Prevention from the DHSS Advisory Committee on Alcoholism, and of the World Health Organisation Expert Committee which in 1980 reported on problems related to alcohol consumption. We support the suggestions of those committees, but, as we hope to show, the implications of this point of view need to be spelled out more clearly.

The need for visible goals

It is more emotionally satisfying and often more engaging of public sympathies and national energies when an attack can be made on a social problem with the battle cry that, if only we attack with sufficient vigour and resolve, the problem can be absolutely rooted out. Issues such as the slave traffic or smallpox could engender an enormous campaigning commitment, both nationally and internationally. Heroin addiction is a contemporary example. Society has no real prospect of totally eliminating alcohol problems. In the absence of any such clear and absolute aim there is inevitable confusion as to the policy goals that should actually be pursued. The evidence presented in Chapter 7 must be taken as firmly supporting the view that the level and manner in which a country uses alcohol will be related to the scale of the damage which alcohol will inflict on that country. Per capita consumption and the ill effects of drinking rise and fall together.

It is easily forgotten that prohibition was once mooted in this country, but today it would be politically inconceivable to inflict that degree of control on the individual pursuit of pleasure, and would imply an unacceptable degree of paternalism. If the United States Prohibition experiment is relevant, it also seems likely that an attempt to ban alcohol in a society which widely desires this substance would lead to a criminally organized black market. Not only is alcohol a source of pleasure which our society would be unwilling to surrender, but is also a source of profit, employment and tax revenue on a huge scale. The production, marketing, and selling of alcoholic beverages employs in excess of three-quarters of a million people. Exports of alcohol exceed £1,000 million a year and amount to nearly 2 per cent of all United Kingdom exports. In 1985 the excise duties and VAT raised on the sale of alcoholic beverages exceeded £5,900 million, about one-third of the cost of running the National Health Service. Understandably there is conflict over the response to drinking problems.

Even in the absence of such political and economic arguments, prohibition would not be any part of our recommendations. Moderate alcohol consumption at an appropriate time and place does not cause harm and for many people it considerably enhances their enjoyment of life. In small quantities it may even reduce the risk of certain forms of heart disease. Alcohol also facilitates relaxation and creates an ambience in which friendship rather than anxiety and mistrust can flourish. Alcohol, unlike tobacco, is not a substance without which we would all be better off.

If alcohol use at both a personal and community level is to be a matter of balancing costs with benefits, what level of harm are we to accept as tolerable? This is a practical question of much human interest which must be brought more into the open. Is the country willing to say that on this or that index of harm (cirrhosis deaths, perhaps, or hospital admissions for alcohol dependence) the increase has been intolerable, that it must be made to reverse the trend? It is the 'targetlessness' of society's present policies on alcohol problems that guarantees failure. One remedy would be to propose that certain definite goals be set up and publicly acknowledged by the government. When concrete intentions have been publicly stated, progress can be effectively monitored.

As a simple set of first-level goals there should be commitment to:

- **Preventing the national per capita alcohol consumption from rising beyond the present level.**

- **Preventing a further rise in any of the available indices of alcohol-related harm – such as liver cirrhosis death rate, drunkenness and drunk driving offences, and hospital admissions for alcohol dependence.**

It might further be suggested that, as a minimal second-stage set of goals, some agreement should be reached as to the level to which alcohol consumption and indices of harm should be brought down over the next decade. We are reluctant to propose definite targets at this stage, acknowledging that such targets can only be set on the basis of consultation and public debate, informed by a knowledge of facts. For example, it might be accepted that the population did not feel itself grossly deprived of drinking opportunities twenty years ago, and it might be an agreed goal to bring the national alcohol consumption back to that previous level, a reduction of approximately one-third. Any chosen goal is arbitrary: the criteria established must certainly take account of political feasibility.

Prevention and government policy

Alcohol-related problems are in many ways a test case for the ability of the administrative structure to tackle complex problems which cross orthodox boundaries. Fifteen different government departments in England and Wales have some concern with alcohol, its benefits and problems, at some stage in its production, distribution, sale, taxation, legislation, and management. The Home Office and DHSS have some responsibility for the drunkenness offender; the Department of the Environment has produced a report on drunk driving; the Home Office set up a Committee on Liquor Licensing; taxation is a matter for the Treasury. The Ministry of Agriculture, Food, and Fisheries has a basic concern with the production of many of the raw materials concerned and is administratively responsible for the alcohol industry. Education in schools is within the purview of the Department of Education and Science. In Scotland and Northern Ireland there are further departments which replicate some of these areas of responsibility. It would be difficult to find any department which is not in some way involved with questions related to alcohol or alcohol problems. Only on the basis of concerted planning is it possible to envisage society dealing effectively with a problem of these protean manifestations, and able continually to evolve policies that can respond to changing conditions and knowledge. Any recommendations in this Report must be sensitive to the working methods of others. With that proviso we would recommend that:

- **Urgent attention be given to improving consultation and working co-operation between different government departments to ensure an integrated, effective, and visible response to the country's drinking problems and their interrelatedness.**

Further recommendations on prevention policies stem directly from the discussion of causes of harmful drinking in Chapter 7. Recognizing the clear association between the price of alcohol and consumption we recommend that:

- **Government taxation policies should be intentionally employed in the interest of health, to ensure that per capita alcohol consumption does not increase beyond the present level, and is by stages brought back to an agreed lower level.**

Increased availability of alcohol is usually associated with a rise in consumption and consequent problems. The number of liquor outlets in the United Kingdom has increased enormously in recent years with the growth in the number of sales outlets in supermarkets and off licences. More than 30,000 new licences have been issued in the past ten years. The past decade has seen a steep rise in licences granted to clubs where drink is substantially cheaper than elsewhere. These changes have been associated with a time of steeply rising consumption but it is likely that price and prosperity have played the main part in this rise and it is extremely difficult to parcel out the contribution which other increases in availability have contributed to this trend. It was observed that the modest increase in permitted hours, an hour in the evenings along with Sunday opening, which came to Scotland in 1976, has had no demonstrable effect on alcohol-related problems.

Although drunkenness offences have fallen since that time, changes in police policy and a worsening economic situation have confused the picture so that the impact of this measure alone cannot be assessed. We think it would be unwise to interpret these findings as justifying an open-all-hours policy for public houses. The evidence of our history and of other countries suggests that we would regret such a move. There has even been a recent move to sell alcohol at petrol stations. We recommend that:

- **The public health implications of measures which increase the availability of alcohol should always be carefully considered and the impact of changes regularly monitored.**

We also recommend further investment in preventive approaches through change in the cultural attitudes which influence drinking. Health education in this area hitherto has had disappointingly little impact. Facile attempts to influence deeply-held cultural beliefs cannot be expected to succeed. This field of endeavour is much in need of imaginative ideas, with an emphasis on concrete behaviours rather than generalities, and studies which allow reliable measurement of outcome. We therefore recommend that:

- **There should be a greatly enhanced government commitment towards public information and education (and relevant evaluative research), so as to bring about a reduction in drinking problems.**

It may also be useful to make some preliminary recommendations as to the general content of the educational messages:

- **Education on alcohol directed to the general public should:**

(a) Keep providing the basic factual knowledge needed to inform public debate in order to win general acceptance of the need for a broad range of preventive measures. The fact that alcohol is a drug and the dose contained in each drink should be made widely known, so should the meaning and implications of dependence, the nature and extent of the toxic effects of alcohol, the dangers of harm to others, and the causes of harmful drinking. In particular, the relationship between national per capita consumption and the extent of the country's drinking problems should be brought repeatedly to public attention.

(b) Convince people that the use of alcohol or other drugs in the attempt to relieve unpleasant feelings when they are apprehensive, dejected, depressed, lonely, or bored, carries considerable risks.

(c) Encourage public disapproval of intoxication, and foster the attitude that it is bad manners to get drunk (rather than that it is bad manners to comment on drunkenness).

(d) Emphasize the dangers and immorality of drinking and driving.

(e) Publicize the risks of mixing drink with other drugs.

(f) Give clear information about the way in which personal risk increases as alcohol consumption rises (see below).

(g) Make clear that persuading guests to drink excessively is not a hallmark of successful hospitality but the reverse (Chapter 9).

(h) Make the workplace a more prominent locus for alcohol education.

Levels of consumption

Providing guidelines as to what constitutes safe, or dangerous, levels of drinking presents particular problems for health education. There is an urgent need for sensible guidelines and yet these often end up by being misinterpreted and misused, for instance, by suggesting that there is a cut-off point below which all drinking is 'safe' and above which it suddenly becomes 'unsafe'. In fact in relation to most alcohol-related problems we are usually dealing with a gradient in which, except at very low levels of consumption, each extra drink adds that little bit more to the personal risk of suffering some harmful consequence.

When our principal concern is the health of the community, the overall aim should be to reduce per capita consumption across the board. *Paradoxically, moderate drinkers, because they are relatively so numerous, make the major contribution to the overall level of alcohol problems in a population* (p. 110). Although heavy drinkers individually carry a greatly increased risk of harm, numerically they represent a minority of drinkers, and therefore collectively still contribute a relatively smaller sum of problems to the community than the total of problems generated by more modest imbibers. One sobering consequence of this is the fact that a very significant reduction in the overall level of harm in the community could be achieved if every drinker among us were to decide to reduce his or her consumption by one-third of its present level.

Many individuals are primarily interested to know their personal risk at different levels of consumption. It is absolutely essential that any individual drinker, educator, or journalist who is concerned about sensible limits for himself, his audience, or readers should first ponder the following commonsense qualifications which must precede any attempt to specify quantities that may be regarded as 'safe' or 'dangerous'. Any final decision on the part of an individual represents a trade-off between the benefits of drinking against the risks of specific hazards. It is worth rehearsing the issues at stake here, although most have been mentioned already in this book.

The pattern of drinking

The way in which any total daily quantity is spaced out is important. Obviously an excessive intake even on a single occasion may result in intoxication, which in certain circumstances can lead, for example, to an accident or to behaviour which is out of character and results in damage to a relationship. There is obviously a big difference between an individual who takes twenty standard drinks on one occasion and the individual who spreads the same number out throughout the week. *On the other hand, regular drinkers who imbibe steadily over many years may develop liver damage or physical dependence without any evident intoxication having ever occurred.*

Context of drinking

Someone, for example, who drinks before driving or operating machinery or looking after a child obviously runs a much greater risk of harmful consequences than the individual who drinks excessively at a party but arranges for a friend to take him home. Where we drink and with whom is obviously important in minimizing or maximizing the chance of harmful consequences.

Physical factors

Physical attributes of the drinker also need to be taken into account. Their weight is obviously important – the lower the weight, the greater the effect of a single dose of alcohol. There is also inbuilt biological variation which to a certain extent protects some individuals against ill effects such as liver cirrhosis and makes others more vulnerable. For instance, some individuals with a family history of alcohol problems are particularly vulnerable to developing alcohol dependence. The greater vulnerability of women and the importance of avoiding heavy drinking in pregnancy have been mentioned in earlier chapters. At the extremes of youth and old age alcohol may have disproportionate effects. The presence of other drugs or illnesses further complicates an already complex picture.

With all the above caveats borne firmly in mind we would join with the

Health Education Council in recommending that the levels of consumption shown in Figure 8 represent a reasonable guide.

For pregnant women either abstinence or minimal consumption of one or two drinks once or twice a week is recommended. In Britain at present between 15 and 20 per cent of men and 1 per cent of women admit to drinking at the 'harmful' level.

The limits recommended here are somewhat more stringent than those previously advised by the College.

Some comment is needed on the expected pay-off from each of these recommendations for a health education agenda. The simple provision of information cannot be expected by itself to influence drinking behaviour or related problems, but it is relevant to building the climate of informed opinion on which so much else may depend. This information is as much for administrators, Members of Parliament, journalists, and the professions as for the population at large. The message given by the individual doctor or teacher, the position taken by a neighbour, the way in which the next television play is presented or the next novel is written, and the attitudes of other

Figure 8   'Drinking guidelines'

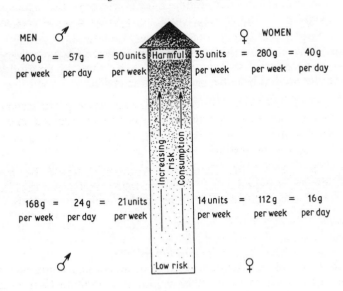

Note: For pregnant women abstinence or minimal consumption is recommended

more immediate and personal educators or agents of change may thus be influenced or given support.

Advertising

The enormous amount of money being spent on liquor advertising has already been noted. It is difficult to determine whether this weight of advertising merely encourages brand switching, or encourages drinking itself. We must all realize that this money is being spent on advertising and marketing a psychoactive and potentially addictive drug. It would be surprising if those thousands of attractive hoardings did not augment the pressures on people to drink. The pervasive images which associate glamour and good times with drinking are fundamentally propaganda for the notion that alcohol is indispensable to the realization of some of our most cherished fantasies. In some countries the advertising of alcohol has been restricted to point of sale only. We are, however, aware of the dangers of too much state interference based on too little evidence, and would here make a provisional recommendation:

- **The government should regularly monitor by means of adequately funded independent research the scale and content of liquor advertising, both direct and indirect, such as sponsorship.**
- **If there is an evident association between such promotions and increases in overall consumption then we recommend that such advertising should be curtailed.**

The voluntary Code of Advertising Practice has a special section on alcohol, but advertisers not infrequently put a lax interpretation on its provisions.

We recommend that:

- **The Advertising Standards Authority should be more clearly independent of the advertising profession itself and we recommend that the code and particularly its implementation should be reviewed.**

Drinking and driving

Convictions for drinking and driving in the United Kingdom have risen from approximately 24,000 in 1967 to 101,000 in 1984. Drunk drivers are responsible for some 1,200 fatalities each year.

It is clear that the law as it stands at present does not deter the drinking driver. Recent estimates suggest that the chances of being caught are only one in 250. The greatest deterrent appears to be not so much the severity of the penalty which can be imposed but the likelihood of detection. We recommend the following steps as urgently necessary if the current level of injury and loss of life is to be reduced:

- **That the Blennerhasset recommendations on discretionary testing should be implemented in an attempt to improve detection rates.**

We regard this change as a priority. Public opinion is now much more critical of the drunk driver and seems ready to accept this development. There is evidence that the introduction of 'random testing' reduced road traffic deaths by 30 per cent in Australia and New Zealand (equivalent to approximately 360 people every year in the United Kingdom).

The public is unaware of the effects of different doses of alcohol on driving skills (pp. 83–4). These should be made more widely known by means of public information campaigns and should be stated in detail in the Highway Code.

A disproportionately large number of drunk driving offences occur among young and inexperienced drivers. In a recent self-report survey one in three young men (age 16–30) admitted that they had driven while over the legal limit and seemed relatively unconcerned about this. A lower permitted limit of blood-alcohol for drivers in the first two years of passing their driving test might help reduce the dangers for inexperienced drivers.

International influences

Increased alcohol consumption in Britain has occurred in the context of a general international trend. The degree of international co-operation which has existed for over half a century as regards trade and trafficking in narcotic drugs, and related monitoring and exchange of information, is in contrast to the nearly non-existent concern with international trade in alcohol. In 1975, however, the World Health Assembly adopted a resolution addressed to member states and to the Director General of the World Health Organisation, calling for the development of monitoring systems for alcohol consumption and other relevant data needed for public health policies on an international scale. The Council of Europe and the European Parliament have recently taken some initiative on health aspects of drinking. The International Council on Alcoholism and Addictions is a voluntary organization which has been actively fostering international collaboration for many years.

Other international agreements may operate to increase consumption, for instance, in Britain as a result of EEC trade agreements. As part of its tax harmonization objectives, the EEC is seeking to equalize the duty ratios on different alcoholic drinks in all member countries and Britain has been accused, and indeed convicted, of operating a tax structure which discriminates against wine. The European Court found against the United Kingdom and the United Kingdom has subsequently acted to alter the ratios of duty on wines and beer. The European Community currently seems preoccupied with harmonizing ratios of duty rather than ratios of price with alcohol content. As a consequence beverages which are relatively cheap to produce will also cost less to the consumer per unit of alcohol. Wine is, therefore, becoming relatively cheaper and as we have seen its consumption is escalating. We therefore recommend that:

- **This country should strongly support initiatives for international recognition of the health and social implications relating to import and export of alcoholic beverages rather than accepting the dominance of the economic interest.**

Impact on employment

Some of the recommendations made here concerning the Government's role in prevention may be regarded as a potential threat to the interests and livelihood of those who have invested their capital in the production of alcohol, or whose livelihood depends on its manufacture, distribution, sale, or advertising. The alcohol industry provides employment for 750,000 people and excise duty on alcohol in 1984 amounted to more than £4,000 million. More than £150 million is spent on the promotion of alcohol. It is none the less evident that unrestrained growth is not compatible with the good health of the community. This Report is concerned with furtherance of health, but its recommendations must also take other important and legitimate interests into account.

- **The possible impact that health-directed policies on alcohol abuse may have on the livelihood of any section of the community should be borne in mind. Those interests should be consulted, and efforts should be made to encourage diversification of investment and facilitate alternative sources of employment.**

Prevention at community and personal level

All levels of prevention interact with one another: government strategies on control or pricing, the methods of health education, and the actions taken by the community. Special efforts must be made to support prevention at the community level, and inherent in the educational message should be an insistence that much of the responsibility lies squarely with the community.

Prevention at community and personal level is best designed in detail by the people immediately concerned. Here are some recommendations:

- Every industrial or commercial undertaking should review the extent to which its employees are under pressure to drink, and then devise means for lessening this pressure. This is especially important where drinking may affect safety.

- Special preventive programmes should be set up for high-risk trades or professions, in collaboration with trades unions or appropriate professional organizations.

- A review should be made in every community of the extent to which leisure activities are available, particularly for the young, that do not engender pressures to drink. Appropriate action should be taken to increase the range of such activities.

- Those responsible for organizing official receptions and similar public functions should serve alcohol only in moderate quantities, and non-alcoholic drinks should always be available. Government and local authorities could set an exemplary role here.

- Those who entertain in their own homes should realize that serving alcohol is a responsibility which cannot be treated casually. Encourage drivers not to drink alcohol and make it easy for them to decline. If guests have become intoxicated ensure that they can get home safely. Non-alcoholic drinks should always be available (Chapter 9).

- Members of the community should not ignore the person who is drinking excessively but should show the same active concern as they would towards any other potentially dangerous behaviour.

- Every person should accept responsibility for his or her own

**personal prevention programme by not exceeding the daily
intake level suggested above. We have a personal
responsibility to monitor our own drinking and keep in
mind the guidelines to sensible drinking and the issues
discussed in Chapter 9.**

These recommendations point only to a few examples of potentially
fruitful community involvement. Some of the recommendations deal
with small issues (the serving of alcohol at a civic reception for
instance), and it might be objected that such recommendations are
puritanical or rather trivial. But only the sum of a great many small or
symbolic actions within individual communities will slowly change
attitudes.

TREATMENT

A basic assumption

To give treatment its proper context within an awareness of what the
individual may be able to accomplish unaided and of what society's
ordinary and informal processes may be expected to accomplish, we
recommend the following basic assumption about the role of
treatment:

- **Skilled help should be available at an early stage to the
  person with a drinking problem. At the same time the
  capacity of individuals with drinking problems to help
  themselves and modify their own behaviour needs to be
  emphasized, as does the importance of the family and the
  wider society in responding to an individual's excessive
  drinking in a helpful way (Chapter 9).**

The planning of treatment services

Over the last three decades much has been learnt about treatment and
its organization, and this constitutes the essential basis of experience
on which the future of treatment has to build. Whatever the
imperfections in the coverage which services have offered in the past, a
great many people have found their way to treatment, and many have
been helped. A great deal of pretence has got to be swept away before
we can appreciate the limited but vital place which the treatment of
drinking problems should be accorded.

The first recommendation which we make has relevance to the
broad strategy of planning treatment services:

- **National policies on treatment services for alcohol problems**

should be designed in the light of a critical appraisal of:
(a) an accurate survey of existing resources in each region;
(b) the efficacy of particular treatments;
(c) the scale upon which that kind of treatment can be introduced within available resources;
(d) the proportion of people with drinking problems who are likely to avail themselves of help of that kind.

To some extent this is simply to commend the obvious and generally accepted basis of service planning. Although recent history provides instances of policies being evolved on just this type of basis (e.g. the piloting of detoxification centres and the current evaluation of community alcohol teams), it would on the other hand not be at all difficult to cite aspects of service planning which have not followed these simple rules (the expansion of hostel places, for example). Rather than long periods of inaction being followed by a hurried launching of new schemes with 'no time for research' it would be better if services were evolved and researched as elements of a more continual and related process. The lack of DHSS guidelines on the treatment of alcohol problems contrasts strangely with the recent provision of guidelines in the field of drug misuse. The lack of such guidelines imposes serious difficulties for service providers at local level.

We also make two further recommendations:

• Treatment of alcohol-related disabilities should be left within the province of primary level agencies, such as health centres and social work departments, whenever possible.

• There is an important role for specialized services, both for treatment of some patients and for support and training of those generalists who will be dealing with the majority of drinking problems.

These recommendations do not enter into details of service planning, but are intended to support the idea that there is room both for the generalist (general practitioner, social worker, nurse, voluntary worker, for instance) and for specialization (special NHS units, specialized voluntary organizations, and so on). The development of services at a regional level requires joint liaison and planning between health, social work, and non-statutory sectors and interests. A truly collaborative style of planning is more likely to be effective than one which is based on a competitive scramble to hold on to scarce resources.

Professional education

The ability of any profession to make its contribution to the treatment of drinking problems must depend both on willingness to participate and on trained skills. We would therefore propose that:

- **Each of the caring professions should systematically examine the role which its members can play in the prevention and treatment of drinking problems, and review the present adequacy of training to meet these responsibilities, and in the light of such considerations formulate and institute appropriate training.**

This last recommendation is purposely made in general terms. It would be wrong for a report coming from one particular professional body to make detailed proposals as to how any other profession – social work, clinical psychology, nursing, pastoral counselling, to name only a few – should go about the task of reviewing the adequacy of its existing training courses. Some organizations have indeed in recent years already made definite moves on professional education in the field of alcohol problems. Clinical psychologists have, for instance, prepared an excellent report on their own profession's potential contribution to the management of alcohol problems. Nurses have developed post-qualifying courses in addictions. The Central Council for Education and Training in Social Work has supported similar developments and has funded further training of social workers in alcohol problems, for instance at the Alcohol Studies Centre in Paisley. Clearly, there is a very general need for professions to review the way in which they are dealing with drinking problems and to do more than pay lip service to the concept of training in team work and joint planning.

RESEARCH

A strong emphasis on the need for research is implicit in much of this Report. Rather than now setting out a 'shopping list' of research topics, we shall make one general recommendation.

This country devotes pitifully few funds to research into alcohol-related problems. It is a curious fact that support for research is often given in inverse proportion to the morbidity and mortality associated with the condition. This was dramatically illustrated in a recent United States study (Table 13), and the position is very similar in this country.

This leads us to the planning and integration of research. The degree to which research should be centrally planned, or alternatively left to the interests of particular individuals and research centres is, of

Table 13   *Investment health research (US) dollars in relation to economic cost*

disorder	research effort 1978 ($ in millions)	economic cost 1975 ($ in billions)	research dollars per thousand ($ of cost)
alcoholism and alcohol abuse	16	43	0.4
cancer	627	19	30
heart and vascular disease	284	46	6
respiratory disease	69	19	4

Source: Institute of Medicine (1980) *Alcoholism, Alcohol Abuse and Alcohol-Related Problems*. Washington DC: National Academy Press.

course, a question that goes wider than alcohol research. But with alcohol and alcohol-related problems there are a number of considerations that specially support the desirability of planning. Where social investigations are concerned, there is often a need for repeated surveys (repeated monitoring of national drinking patterns, for instance), or a long-term follow-up of particular groups (people with different types of drinking problem or different drinking patterns, the children of excessive drinkers, and so on). There is also often a need to anticipate events: a change in licensing provision or an abrupt change in price should be preceded as well as followed by research.

There is also a general need to find ways of making use of research findings in the development of policies, whether this is in relation to any of the prevention strategies that have been discussed, or in relation to the design of treatment services.

Interdisciplinary research is needed of a type which the structure of university departments does not always encourage. The general question of the need to set priorities applies urgently to alcohol research because resources are inevitably limited, whereas the array of medico-social problems is enormous and pressing. The exchange of scientific information, even on such an obvious topic as who is doing what research, the collation of existing data, and the training of research workers are also matters that should fall within an integrated plan. (A helpful development here has been the periodic listing of ongoing alcohol research compiled by the Alcohol Research Group in Edinburgh.)

The need for planning should be taken seriously as it provides a test case for the scientific policy-making of this country. (A recent promising example was the DHSS homelessness and addictions research liaison group strategy for research on alcoholism.)

We recommend that:

- **Research funding should be commensurate with the social and health costs of alcohol misuse.**

INTO THE FUTURE

Our society has chosen to co-exist with a potentially dangerous and addictive drug. Society must therefore accept responsibility for dealing with the problems that arise, and for as far as possible averting the occurrence of those problems. The helping professions are part of society, and their role and the powers and limitations of what they can offer have to be understood by society.

Society has in many ways tried to savour its pleasure, avoid its responsibilities, and hand the problem over to the courts or the caring agencies. We believe that a vital message for the future is that preventive measures have to be strengthened, and that this will inevitably mean all of us drinking somewhat less than we do at present. We cannot pretend to be concerned while complaining that any diminution of our personal pleasures or profits is too great a price.

Society also needs to deal with its fantasies and its prejudices. People with drinking problems are very much 'of us' – they are not to be put aside as a strange, abhorrent, and disgraced minority. Future action on these problems requires understanding of their pervasiveness in our society and, in every sense, their pain. The damage is vastly greater than that caused by heroin addiction. The problems are complex, and we are still a long way from being able to produce any easy solution. Society should, though, be appalled by the present state of affairs and entirely unwilling to witness continued loss and suffering of this order.

Bibliography

One way of dealing with a bibliography for this Report would have been to provide full references to support every statement made, as would be the usual academic practice. Rather than adopt that academic style, we shall give a relatively brief bibliography of key references, purposely designed to be of practical use to the sort of wide readership we have in mind. There is naturally some overlap between topics in various texts.

GENERAL AND INTRODUCTION (CHAPTER 1)

British Medical Journal (1982) *Alcohol Problems*. London: BMJ Publications.
Collins, J.J. Jnr (ed.) (1982) *Drinking and Crime*. London: Tavistock.
Consumers Association (1984) Alcohol and your health. *Which*, October.
Crawford, A. and Stuart, R. (1986) *Register of Alcohol Research in the United Kingdom, 1985–1986*. London: Brewers' Society.
Heather, N. and Robertson, I. (1986) *Problem Drinking*. Pelican Books.
Madden, J.S. (1979) *A Guide to Alcohol and Drug Dependence*. Bristol: Wright and Sons.
Plant, M.A. (ed.) (1982) *Drinking and Problem Drinking*. London: Junction Books: Fourth Estate.
Plant, M.A. (1986) *Drugs in Perspective*. London: Hodder and Stoughton.
Raistrick, D. and Davidson, R. (1986) *Alcoholism and Drug Dependence*. London: Churchill Livingstone.
Walls, H.J. and Brownlie, A.R. (1983) *Drink, Drugs and Crime*. London: Sweet and Maxwell.

HISTORICAL TRENDS (CHAPTER 2)

Berridge, V. (1977) Opium and the historical perspective. *Lancet* ii: 78–80.
Berridge, V. and Edwards, G. (1981) *Opium and the People*. London: Allen Lane.
Edwards, G. (1971) *Unreason in an Age of Reason*. London: Royal Society of Medicine.

Encyclopaedia Britannica (15th edn.) (1975) Text article on alcohol consumption (by M. Keller).

Smart, R.G. (1974) The effect of licencing restrictions during 1914–18 on drunkenness and liver cirrhosis deaths in Britain. *British Journal of Addiction* 69: 109–21.

Spring, J.A. and Buss, D.H. (1977) Three centuries of alcohol in the British diet. *Nature* 270: 567–72.

Porter, R. (1985) The drinking man's disease: the 'pre-history' of alcoholism in Georgian Britain. *British Journal of Addiction* 80: 385–96.

PRESENT PERSPECTIVES (CHAPTER 3)

Advisory Committee on Alcoholism (1979) *Report on Education and Training.* DHSS and Welsh Office. London: HMSO.

Camberwell Council on Alcoholism (1980) *Women and Alcohol.* London: Tavistock.

Central Policy Review Staff (1979) *Alcohol Policies in the United Kingdom.* Stockholm: Sociologists Institutionen, Stockholm Universitet.

Department of the Environment (1976) *Drinking and Driving: Report of the Departmental Committee* (Blennerhasset). London: HMSO.

Department of Health and Social Security (1978) *The Pattern and Range of Services for Problem Drinkers: Report by the Advisory Committee on Alcoholism.* London: HMSO.

Department of Health and Social Security (1981) *Drinking Sensibly.* London: HMSO.

Detoxification Evaluation Project (1985) *Problem Drinking: Experiments in Detoxification.* London: Bedford/NCVO.

Home Office (1971) *Habitual Drinker Offenders.* London: HMSO.

Moser, J. (1985) *Alcohol Policies in National Health and Development Planning.* Offset Publication 89. Geneva: World Health Organization.

United States Department of Health and Human Services (1983) *Alcohol and Health.* Washington: National Institute on Alcohol Abuse and Alcoholism.

ALCOHOL AND ITS EFFECTS (CHAPTER 4)

Rosalki, S. (ed.) (1984) *Clinical Biochemistry of Alcoholism.* London: Churchill Livingstone.

Wallgren, H. and Barry, H. (1970) *Actions of alcohol. Vol. 1: Biochemical, Physiological and Psychological Aspects.* Amsterdam: Elsevier.

CONCEPTS OF DEPENDENCE (CHAPTER 5)

Edwards, G. and Cross, M.M. (1976) Alcohol dependence syndrome. Provisional description of a clinical syndrome. *British Medical Journal* 1: 1058–061.

Heather, N., Robertson, I., and Davies, P. (1985). *The Misuse of Alcohol.* London: Croom Helm.

Hodgson, R., Stockwell, T., Rankin, H., and Edwards, G. (1978) Alcohol

dependence: the concept its utility and measurement. *British Journal of Addiction* 73: 339–42.
World Health Organisation (1977) *Alcohol Related Disabilities*. Offset Publication 32. Geneva: World Health Organisation.

ALCOHOL-RELATED DISABILITIES (CHAPTER 6)

Hore, B.D. (1976) *Alcohol dependence*. London: Butterworth.
Hore, B.D. and Plant, M.A. (eds) (1981) *Alcohol Problems in Employment*. London: Croom Helm.
McDonnell, R. and Maynard, A. (1985) The Costs of Alcohol Misuse. *British Journal of Addiction* 80: 27–36.
Orford, J. and Harwin, J. (eds) (1982) *Alcohol and the Family*. London: Croom Helm.
Plant, M.L. (1985) *Women, Drinking and Pregnancy*. London: Tavistock.
Rosett, H.L. and Weiner, L. (1984) *Alcohol and the Fetus*. New York; Oxford University Press.
Sherlock, S. (ed.) (1982) Alcohol and Disease. *British Medical Bulletin* 38. London: Churchill Livingstone.
Tygstrup, N. and Olsson, R. (eds) (1986) *Acta Medica Scandinavica Symposium Series No. 1*. Stockholm: Almquist and Wiksell International.

SOCIAL CAUSES OF HARMFUL DRINKING (CHAPTER 7)

Bruun, K., Lumio, M., Mäkela, K., Pan, L., Popham, R.E., Room, R., Schmidt, W., Skog, O., Sulkunnen, P., and Osterberg, E. (1975) *Alcohol Control Policies in Public Health Perspective*. Helsinki: Finnish Foundation for Alcohol Studies.
Grant, M., Plant, M.A., and Williams, A. (eds) (1983) *Economics and Alcohol*. London: Croom Helm.
Kendell, R.E. (1985) The determinants of per capita consumption. In *Alcohol: Preventing the Harm*. London: Institute of Alcohol Studies.
Kendell, R.E., de Roumanie, M. and Ritson, E.B. (1983) Effect of economic changes on Scottish drinking habits 1978–82. *British Journal of Addiction* 78: 365–79.
McGuinness, T. (1979) *An Econometric Analysis of Total Demand for Alcoholic Beverages in the UK, 1965–75*. Edinburgh: Scottish Health Education Unit.
Nielsen, J. and Sorensen, K. (1979) Alcohol policy: alcohol consumption, alcohol prices, delirium tremens and alcoholism as cause of death in Denmark. *Social Psychiatry* 14: 133–38.
Spring, J.A. and Buss, D.H. (1977) Three centuries of alcohol in the British diet. *Nature* 270: 567–72.
Wald, I. and Moskalewicz, J. (1984) Alcohol policy in a crisis situation. *British Journal of Addiction* 79: 331–35.

INDIVIDUAL CAUSES OF HARMFUL DRINKING (CHAPTER 8)

Goodwin, D. (1976) *Is Alcoholism Hereditary?* New York: Oxford University Press.

National Institute on Alcohol Abuse and Alcoholism (1983) *Biological/Genetic Factors in Alcoholism*. Washington DC: DHHS.
Orford, J. (1985) *Excessive Appetites*. Chichester: John Wiley.

PERSONAL RESPONSIBILITY AND SELF-HELP (CHAPTER 9)

Chick, J. and Chick, J. (1984) *Drinking Problems with Advice and Information for the Individual Family and Friends*. London: Churchill Livingstone.
Grant, M. (1984) *Same Again*. Harmondsworth: Penguin.
Robertson, I. and Heather, N. (1986) *Let's Drink to your Health: A Self-help Guide to Healthier Drinking*. Leicester: British Psychological Society.

TREATMENT FOR PROBLEM DRINKERS (CHAPTER 10)

Edwards, G. (1982) *Treatment of Drinking Problems*. London: Grant McIntyre.
Edwards, G. and Grant, M. (1980) *Alcoholism Treatment and Transition*. London: Croom Helm.
Orford, J. and Edwards, G. (1977) *Alcoholism*. Oxford: Oxford University Press.
Robertson, I. and Heather, N. (1981) *Controlled Drinking*. London: Methuen.
Robertson, I., Hodgson, R., Orford, J., and McKechnie, R. (1984) *Psychology and Problem Drinking*. London: British Psychological Society.
Robinson, D. (1979) *Talking Out of Alcoholism*. London: Croom Helm.
Shaw, S., Cartwright, A., Spratley, T., and Harwin, J. (1978) *Responding to Drinking Problems*. London: Croom Helm.
Skinner, H.A. and Holt, S. (1983) Early intervention for alcohol problems. *Journal of the Royal College of General Practitioners* 33: 787–91.
Vaillant, G. (1983) *The Natural History of Alcoholism*. London: Harvard University Press.
Zimberg, S., Wallace, J., and Blume, S. (1978) *Practical Approaches to Alcoholism Psychotherapy*. New York: Plenum.

PREVENTIVE AND FUTURE POLICIES (CHAPTER 11)

Grant, M. and Ritson, B. (1983) *Alcohol: The Prevention Debate*. London: Croom Helm.
Grant, M., Plant, M., and Williams, A. (eds) (1983) *Economics and Alcohol*. London: Croom Helm.
Plant, M.A., Peck, D., and Samuel, E. (1985) *Alcohol, Drugs and School Leavers*. London: Tavistock.
Ross, H.L. (1982) *Deterring the Drinking Driver*. Lexington: Lexington Books.
Singler, E. and Storm, T. (eds) (1985) *Public Drinking and Public Policy*. Toronto: Addiction Research Foundation.
Tether, P. and Robinson, D. (1986) *Preventing Alcohol Problems*. London: Tavistock.
Walsh, B. and Grant, M. (1985) *Public Health Implications of Alcohol Production and Trade*. Offset Publication 88. Geneva: World Health Organisation.

World Health Organisation (1980) *Problems Related to Alcohol Consumption*. Technical Report Series. Geneva: World Health Organisation.
World Health Organisation (1985) *Alcohol Policies*. Report Publication, European Series 18. Geneva: World Health Organisation.

Appendix
Useful sources
of help and information
(compiled by
Ray Stuart,
Alcohol Research Group)

SOURCES OF INFORMATION

Alcohol Concern,
305 Gray's Inn Road, LONDON WC1X 8QF (01-833-3471)
Health Education Council,
78 New Oxford Street, LONDON WC1 1AH (01-637-1881)
Medical Council on Alcoholism,
1 St Andrews Place, LONDON NW1 4LB (01-487-4445)
Northern Ireland Council on Alcohol,
40 Elmwood Avenue, BELFAST BT9 6AZ (0232-664434)
Scottish Council on Alcohol,
147 Blythswood Street, GLASGOW G2 4EN (041-333-9677)
Scottish Health Education Group,
Woodburn House, Canaan Lane, EDINBURGH EH10 4SG (031-447-8044)

AGENCIES HELPING WITH ALCOHOL PROBLEMS

Action on Alcohol Abuse,
26 Craven Street, LONDON WC2 5NT (01-839-7344/5)

Alcoholics Anonymous,
PO Box 514, 11 Redcliffe Gardens, LONDON SW10 9BQ
(01-352-9779/5493)

Al-Anon Family Groups,
61 Great Dover Street, LONDON SE1 4YF (01-403-0888)

Al-Ateen, which caters for the children of problem drinkers, can also be contacted on 01-403-0888.

Drinkwatchers,
200 Seagrave Road, LONDON SW6 1RQ (01-381-3155)

Drugs, Alcohol, Women, Nationally – DAWN
Boundary House, 91–93 Charterhouse Street, LONDON, EC1M 6HR
(01-250-3284)

Teachers Advisory Council on Alcohol and Drug Education
(TACADE),
2 Mount Street, MANCHESTER M2 5NG (061-834-7210)

Turning Point,
CAP House, 9/12 Long Lane, LONDON EC1A 9HA (01-606-3947)

Women's Alcohol Centre,
254 St Paul's Road, Islington, LONDON N1 (01-226-4581)

Accept,
Western Clinic, Seagrave Road, LONDON SW6 1RZ (01-381-3155)

Accept,
Broadway Clinic, The Broadway (off Montrose Road), WIELDSTONE,
Middlesex HA3 7EH (01-427-7700)

Accept,
Parkway Health Centre, Parkway, WELWYN GARDEN CITY, Hertfordshire
(07073-32157)

Accept,
Royal Hospital, Kewfoot Road, RICHMOND UPON THAMES, Surrey TW10
(01-940-7452)

Accept,
Clerks Croft Hospital, Tandridge Day Unit, BLETCHINGLEY, Surrey
(0883-843823)

Accept,
170a Heston Road, Heston, HOUNSLOW, Middlesex (01-577-6059)

EIRE

Al-Anon Information Centre,
12 Westmorland Street, DUBLIN 4 Eire (0001-774195)

Alcoholics Anonymous (Eire),
Service Office, 26 Essex Way, DUBLIN (0001-774809)
The Irish National Council on Alcoholism (for Eire),
19–20 Fleet Street, DUBLIN 2 (0001-774832)

NORTHERN IRELAND

Alcoholics Anonymous (AA),
Central Services Office, 152 Lisburn Road, BELFAST BT9 6AJ
(0232-681084)
Al-Anon,
Information Office, 64 Donegall Street, BELFAST BT1 2GT (0232-243489)
Al-Ateen,
Information Office (as above)
Council on Alcohol-Related Problems,
12 Lombard Street, BELFAST (0232-224176)

SCOTLAND

Alcoholics Anonymous,
50 Wellington Street, GLASGOW G2 (041-221-9027)
Al-Anon Information Centre,
Room 13, 136 Ingram Street, GLASGOW G1 1EJ (041-552-2828)
Alcohol Studies Centre,
Westerfield Annexe, 25 High Calside, PAISLEY PA2 6BY (041-889-3225)
(041-887-1241, Extn 359)
Drinkwatchers,
Edinburgh University, Royal Edinburgh Hospital, EDINBURGH, EH10 5HF
(031-447-2011)

ENGLAND

Local Councils on alcoholism and alcohol advisory services
Avon Council on Alcoholism,
14 Park Row, BRISTOL BS1 5LJ (0272-293028/9)
Berkshire Council on Alcoholism,
342 Oxford Road, READING RG3 1AF (0734-598850)
Birmingham Alcohol Advisory Service,
32 Essex Street, BIRMINGHAM B5 4TR (021-622-2041)
Buckinghamshire Council on Alcoholism,
Tindal Cottage, Bierton Road, AYLESBURY, Bucks HP20 1EW
(0296-25329)

Cambridgeshire Alcohol Advisory Service,
1 Wentworth Street, PETERBOROUGH PE1 1DH (0733-47105)

Cleveland and South Durham Council on Alcoholism,
Albert Centre, 3 Albert Terrace, MIDDLESBROUGH, Cleveland TS1 3PA
(0642-221484)

Cornwall Council on Alcoholism,
The Cornish Unit Building, 14 High Cross Street, ST AUSTELL, Cornwall
(0726-73984)

Coventry Alcohol Advisory Service,
5a Priory Row, COVENTRY CV1 5EX (0203-26619/26610)

Cumbria Alcohol Advisory Service,
Croft House, Wigton Road, CARLISLE CA2 7EP (0228-44140)

Derby Alcohol Problems Advisory Service (DAPAS)
1a College Place, DERBY DE1 3DY (0332-45537)

Devon Council on Alcoholism,
59 Centre, 59 Magdalen Street, EXETER EX2 4HY (0392-55151)

Doncaster Agency on Alcohol Misuse,
28 Copley Road, DONCASTER, South Yorkshire (0302-68705)

East Sussex Alcohol Information Centre,
190 Church Road, HOVE, Sussex (0273-739147) (0424-223850)

Essex Alcohol Advisory Service,
11 Centurion House, St John's Street, COLCHESTER CO2 7AH
(0206-575810)

Gloucestershire Alcohol Information Centre,
23 St George's Road, CHELTENHAM GL51 7DB (0242-584881)

Grimsby Alcohol Counselling Centre,
19 Dudley Street, GRIMSBY (0472-40001)

Hampshire Alcohol Advice Centre,
147 Shirley Road, SOUTHAMPTON (0703-30219)

Hereford and Worcester Alcohol Advisory Service,
10 Sansome Place, WORCESTER WR1 1UA (0905-27417)

Hertfordshire and Bedfordshire Alcohol Problems Advisory Service,
6a Bute Street, LUTON LU1 2BE (0582-23434)

Huddersfield, Unit 51
1st Floor, 24 Westgate, HUDDERSFIELD HD1 1NU (0484-510826)

Humberside Council on Alcoholism,
St Andrew's Information and Advisory Centre, Albion Street,
GRIMSBY DN32 7DY (0472-53416)

Kent Council on Alcoholism,
41 Wincheap, CANTERBURY, Kent (0227-454740)

Leeds Council on Alcoholism,
21/22 West Bar Chambers, 38 Boar Lane, LEEDS LS1 5DB (0532-31029)

Leicestershire Alcohol Advisory Service,
Meetu House, 70 London Road, LEICESTER LE2 0QD (0533-552212)

Lincolnshire Counselling Service for Problem Drinkers and Their Families,
Upper Ground Floor, Viking House, Newland, LINCOLN LN1 1XY
(0522-21908)

Greater London Alcohol Advisory Service,
91–3 Charterhouse Street, LONDON EC1M 6BT (01-253-6221)

Greater Manchester and Lancashire Council on Alcoholism,
87 Oldham Street, MANCHESTER M4 1LN (061-834-9777)

Merseyside, Lancashire and Cheshire Council on Alcoholism,
The Fruit Exchange, Victoria Street, LIVERPOOL L2 6QU
(051-236-0300/1372)

Milton Keynes Alcohol Project,
The David Baxter Centre, 63 North Seventh Street, CENTRAL MILTON
KEYNES MK9 2DP (0908-6633427)

Norfolk Community Alcohol Service,
11 Parsonage Square, NORWICH (0603-660070)

Northampton Alcohol Counselling and Information Service,
24 Hazelwood Road, NORTHAMPTON NN1 1LN (0604-22121)

North Derbyshire Alcohol Advice Centre,
55 Vicars Lane, CHESTERFIELD (0246-206514)

North East Council on Addictions,
1 Mosley Street, NEWCASTLE-UPON-TYNE NE1 1YE (0632-320797)

North Yorkshire Council on Alcoholism,
10 Priory Street, YORK YO1 1EZ (0904-52104)

Nottinghamshire Alcohol Problems Advisory Service,
APAS House, Mount Street, NOTTINGHAM NG1 6HE (0602-414747)

Oxfordshire Council on Alcoholism,
c/o Health Education Unit, 103 Banbury Road, OXFORD OX2 6JZ
(0865-511451)

Plymouth Alcohol Advisory Council,
c/o Plymouth Regional Health Authority, 7 Nelson Gardens,
PLYMOUTH PL1 5RH (0752-52552)

Portsmouth Alcohol Advice Centre,
All Saints Church, Commercial Road, PORTSMOUTH, Hants.
(0705-735911)

Scunthorpe Council on Alcoholism,
48 Oswald Road, SCUNTHORPE DN15 7PQ (0724-854763)

Sheffield Alcohol Advisory Service,
646 Abbeydale Road, SHEFFIELD 7 (0742-587553)

Somerset Council on Alcoholism,
3 Upper High Street, TAUNTON, Somerset TA1 3PX (0823-88174)

Thamesdown and North Wiltshire Council on Alcoholism,
13 Bath Road, SWINDON, Wilts SNL 4AS (0793-695405)

West Dorset Council on Alcoholism,
28 High West Street, DORCHESTER, Dorset DT1 1XF (0305-65901)

WALES

Clwyd and Gwynedd Council on Alcoholism,
Eryl Wen, Eryl Place, LLANDUDNO (0492-76841)

Dyfed Council on Alcoholism,
1 Penlan Road, CARMARTHEN, Dyfed (0267-231634)

Gwent Council on Alcohol and Drug Abuse,
Emlyn House, 3 Palmyra Place, NEWPORT, Gwent NPT 4EJ (0633-63185)

South Glamorgan Council on Alcoholism,
13 Richmond Crescent, CARDIFF (0222-499499)

West Glamorgan Council on Drugs and Alcohol,
75 Uplands Crescent, SWANSEA, West Glamorgan (0792-472519)

CHANNEL ISLANDS

Guernsey Council on Alcoholism,
50 The Bordage, ST PETER PORT, Guernsey, Channel Islands
(0481-23255)

Jersey Council on Alcoholism,
2 Colomberie Chambers, 1 Green Street, ST HELIER, Channel Islands
(0534-26672)

SCOTLAND
Local councils on alcoholism

Borders Council on Alcoholism,
96–98 High Street, GALASHIELS (0896-57657, answering service)

Central Scotland Council on Alcoholism,
c/o Dr C. J. M. Bentley, Secretary, Forth Valley Health Board,
33 Spittal Street, STIRLING (0786-63031)

Fife Council on Alcoholism,
30 North Street, GLENROTHES, Fife (0592-759543)

Alcoholism Information Centre,
Aberdeen and District Council on Alcoholism, 443 Union Street, ABERDEEN
(0224-573887)

Moray Council on Alcoholism,
Alcohol Information Centre, 80 High Street, ELGIN IV30 2NW
(0343-45959)

Caithness Council on Alcoholism,
c/o Social Work Department, Bridge Street, WICK KW1 4AB
(0955-3761, Extn 290)

Inverness Council on Alcoholism,
106 Church Street, INVERNESS (0463-220995)

Lochaber Council on Alcoholism,
c/o Mrs S. Forbes, Secretary, 5 Glenkingle Street, Caol, FORT WILLIAM
(0397-3343)

Ross and Cromarty Council on Alcoholism,
8 High Street, ALNESS, Easter Ross (0349-882249, 24-hour answering
service, cleared daily)

The Council on Alcoholism for Skye and Lochalsh,
Advice and Information Centre, The Green, PORTREE, Isle of Skye
(0478-2633, 24-hour answering machine)

Edinburgh and District Council on Alcoholism,
24 Ainslie Place, EDINBURGH EH3 6AJ (031-226 4519)

Orkney Council on Alcoholism,
4 Warrens Walk, KIRKWALL, Orkney KW15 1DX (0856-4738)

Ayrshire Council on Alcoholism,
2 Bridge Lane, KILMARNOCK (0563-41155)

Bute Council on Alcoholism,
c/o Mrs N. A. Mackenzie, Secretary, 76 Ardbeg Road, ROTHESAY
(0700-4990)

Clydebank and District Council on Alcoholism,
Stirling House, 1 Mill Road, CLYDEBANK (041-952-0996) (0389-73319)
(041-952-4200)

Cowal Council on Alcoholism,
c/o Mrs F. Frow, Secretary, Woodbank, INNELLAN, Argyle PA23 7SB
(036-983-547)

Dumbarton District Council on Alcoholism,
West Bridgend Lodge, West Bridgend, DUMBARTON (0389-31456)

Glasgow Council on Alcoholism,
82 West Regent Street (1st Floor), GLASGOW G2 (041-33-9111)

Inverclyde Council on Alcoholism,
4 Brymner Street, GREENOCK, Renfrewshire (0475-85695)

Islay Council on Alcoholism,
Claddach Centre, Shore Street, BOWMORE, Isle of Islay
(049-681-484, daytime) (049-681-226, Thursday 7–9 p.m.)

Kintyre Council on Alcoholism,
Castlehill, CAMPBELLTOWN, Argyll (0586–53555)

East Kilbride District Council on Alcoholism,
c/o Mrs L. Gauld, Secretary, 2 Glen Quoich, St Leonards, EAST KILBRIDE
(03552-26341)

Mid-Argyll Council on Alcoholism,
1 Argyll Street, LOCHGILPHEAD (0546-2880)

Douglas Association (Monklands Council on Alcoholism), Advice
Centre on Alcohol,
81c Hallcraig Street, AIRDRIE ML6 6AN (02364-53341/53263)

Oban and Lorn Council on Alcoholism,
90 George Street, OBAN, Argyll (0631-65156)

Renfrew District Council on Alcoholism,
Community Service Centre (formerly St Mary's School), Queen Street,
PAISLEY PA1 2TU (041-887-0880) (041-889-1061)

Tayside Area Council on Alcoholism, Alcohol Advice and Information
Centre,
132a Nethergate, DUNDEE DD1 4ED (0382-23965)

ALCOHOL TREATMENT UNITS IN OR ATTACHED TO HOSPITALS

England

London Area

Alcoholism Unit,
The Maudsley Hospital, Denmark Hill, LONDON SE5 8AZ
(01-703-6333)

Alcoholism Unit,
St Bernard's Hospital, Uxbridge Road, SOUTHALL, Middlesex
(01-843-0736)

Elmdene ATU,
Bexley Hospital, Old Bexley Lane, BEXLEY, Kent DA5 2BW (0322-526282)

Cambridgeshire

Drinking Problem Clinic,
Fulbourne Hospital, CAMBRIDGE CB1 5EF (0223-248074)
Drinking Problem Clinic,
Bretton Health Centre, Bretton, PETERBOROUGH, Cambridgeshire
(0733-264506)

Cheshire

Merseyside Regional Alcohol & Drug Dependence Unit,
West Cheshire Hospital, Liverpool Road, CHESTER, Cheshire CH1 3ST
(0244-379333)
Alcoholism Unit,
Moston Hospital, Liverpool Road, CHESTER CH2 4AA (0244-382020)
Priory Unit,
Parkside Hospital, Victoria Road, MACCLESFIELD, Cheshire SK10 2PX
(0625-21000, Extn 376)

Dorset

Herbert Day Hospital,
49 Alumhurst Road, Westbourne, BOURNEMOUTH BH4 8EP
(0202-765-323)

Essex

Alcoholism Treatment Unit,
Larch House, Severalls Hospital, COLCHESTER, Essex
(0206-77271, Extn 67)

Gloucestershire

Coney Hill Hospital,
Coney Hill, GLOUCESTER GL4 7QJ (0452-67033, Extn 230)

Hampshire

Eastleigh Ward,
Basingstoke District Hospital, Psychiatric Division,
BASINGSTOKE RG24 9NA (0256-3202)
Nelson Ward ATU
St James Hospital, PORTSMOUTH PO4 8LD (0705-735211, Extn 249)

Hereford and Worcester

Problem Drinking Unit,
Worcester Royal Infirmary, Newtown Branch, WORCESTER WR5 1JG
(0905-353507)

Humberside

Alcoholic Unit,
Burkhill Ward, Broadgate Hospital, Walkington, BEVERLEY,
Humberside HU17 8RN (0482-868161)

Kent

Longfield House,
Bethlem Royal Hospital, Monks Orchard Road, BECKENHAM, Kent
(01-777-6611)

Mount Zeehan Unit,
St Martins Hospital, Littlebourne Road, CANTERBURY, Kent (0227-61310)

Lancashire

Alcoholism Treatment Unit,
Harvey House, Lancaster Moor Hospital, LANCASTER, Lancashire LA1 3JR
(0524-65241, Extn 216)

Kingswood Clinic,
Prestwick Hospital, MANCHESTER M25 7BL (061-773-9121)

Alcoholism Treatment Unit,
Withington Hospital, West Didsbury, MANCHESTER M20 8LR
(061-445-8111, Extn 2165)

Ward 24, Department of Psychiatry,
North Manchester General Hospital, Delaunays Road, Crumpsall,
MANCHESTER M8 6RB (061-730-1444, Extn 305)

Merseyside

Lakeside Clinic,
Park Day Hospital, Orphan Drive, LIVERPOOL 6 (051-263-2281)

Windsor Clinic,
Rainhill Hospital, PRESCOT, Merseyside (051-426-6511)

Norfolk

Chatterton House,
Goodwins Road, KING'S LYNN, Norfolk PE30 5PD (0553-6626)

St Nicholas Hospital,
Queens Road, GREAT YARMOUTH, Norfolk (0493-57321)

Yare Clinic,
West Norwich Hospital, Bowthorpe Road, NORWICH, Norfolk NR2 3UD
(0603-28377, Extn 8330)

Nottinghamshire

Alcoholism Treatment Unit,
Mapperley Hospital, Porchester Road, NOTTINGHAM NG3 6AA
(0602-608144)

Oxfordshire

The Ley Clinic,
Littlemore Hospital, LITTLEMORE, Oxfordshire (0865-778711, Extn 246)

Somerset

McGarvey Ward,
Mendip Hospital, WELLS, Somerset BA5 3D (0749-72211)
Psychiatric Unit,
Yeovil District Hospital, YEOVIL, Somerset BA21 4AT (0935-5122)

Staffordshire

Weston Villa,
St George's Hospital, Corporation Street, STAFFORD ST16 3AG
(0785-3411, Extn 235)

Surrey

Pinel House,
Regional Alcoholic Unit, Warlingham Park Hospital,
WARLINGHAM CR3 9YR Surrey (08832-2101)
Arnold Scott Unit,
Department of Psychiatry, Epsom District Hospital, Dorking Road, EPSOM,
Surrey (03727-26109)

West Sussex

Sandown House,
Graylingwell Hospital, CHICHESTER, West Sussex PO19 4PQ
(0243-787970, Extn 137)
Crawley Hospital,
West Green Drive, CRAWLEY, West Sussex (0293-27866)
St Francis Hospital,
Colwell Road, HAYWARDS HEATH, West Sussex RH16 4EZ (0444-51881)

Tyne and Wear

Parkwood House Alcohol and Drug Problem Service,
St Nicholas Hospital, Gosforth, NEWCASTLE-UPON-TYNE NE3 3XT
(0632-850151)

Warwickshire

Woodleigh Alcoholism Unit,
Central Hospital, HATTON, Warwickshire CV35 7EE (0926-496241,
Extn 224/257)

Alcoholism Unit,
Central Hospital, HATTON, Warwickshire CB35 7EE (0926-496241)

West Midlands

Regional Drug Addiction & Alcoholism Treatment Unit,
All Saint's Hospital, Lodge Road, BIRMINGHAM B18 5SD (021-523-5151,
Extn 176/108/109)

Psychiatric Unit,
Walsgrave Hospital, Clifford Bridge Road, COVENTRY, West Midlands
(0203-613232)

West Yorkshire

Alcoholism Treatment Unit,
Scalebor Park Hospital, Moor Lane, Burley in Wharfedale, ILKELY,
West Yorkshire LS29 7AJ (09435-2031)

Wales

South Glamorgan

Addiction Treatment & Research Unit,
Ward West 1, Whitchurch Hospital, Whitchurch, CARDIFF CF4 7XB
(0222-62191, Extn 138)

Northern Ireland

Alcohol Treatment Unit,
Ward 15, Downshire Hospital, DOWNPATRICK (0396-33111)

Northlands Centre,
68 Northland Road, LONDONDERRY (0504-263011/268886)

Alcoholism Treatment Unit,
Shaftsbury Square Hospital, Shaftsbury Square, BELFAST (0232-229808)

Holywell Hospital,
ANTRIM BT41 2RJ (084941-5211)

Alcohol Treatment Unit,
Tyrone and Fermanagh Hospital, OMAGH BT79 0NS (0662-45211)

Eire

St Lomain's,
Ballyowen, County Dublin (0001-264077)
St Dympna's,
North Circular Road, Dublin 7 (0001-300105)
St Patrick's Hospital,
James' Street, Dublin 8 (0001-775423)
St Ita's Hospital,
Portrane, County Dublin (0001-450337)

Scotland

Dumfries and Galloway Region

Drinking Problems Unit,
Glencairn Ward, Crichton Royal Hospital, DUMFRIES DG1 4TG
(0387-55301)

Lothian Region

Alcohol Problems Clinic,
Royal Edinburgh Hospital, Morningside Terrace, EDINBURGH EH10 5HF
(031-447-2011)

Strathclyde Region

Dykebar Hospital,
Grahamston Road, PAISLEY PA2 7DE (041-883-5122)
Alcoholism Treatment Unit,
Argyll and Bute Hospital, Lochgilphead, ARGYLL PA31 8LD (0546-2323)
Alcoholism Treatment Unit,
Gartnavel Royal Hospital, 1055 Great Western Road, GLASGOW G12
(041-334-6241)
Alcohol Treatment Unit,
Psychiatric Unit, Monklands District General Hospital, AIRDRIE,
Lanarkshire (02364-69344)
Alcohol Unit,
Ravenscraig Hospital, Inverkip Road, GREENOCK PA16 9HY (0475-29433)
Woodilee Hospital,
Lenzie, GLASGOW G66 3UG (041-776-2451)

Alcohol Clinic,
Southern General Hospital, GLASGOW G51 4TF (041-445-2466)

Alcoholism Treatment Unit,
Hartwood Hospital, SHOTTS, Lanarkshire (0501-20373)

Charing Cross Clinic,
8 Woodside Crescent, GLASGOW G3 7UY (041-332-5463)

Tayside Region

Department of Psychiatry,
Ninewells Medical School, DUNDEE (0382-60111, Extn 2419)

Tayside Area Alcoholism Unit,
Sunnyside Royal Hospital, MONTROSE DD10 9JP (067-483-361)

Royal Dundee Liff Hospital,
DUNDEE DD2 5NF (0328-580441)

Highland Region

Craig Dunain Hospital,
INVERNESS IV3 6JV (0463-34101)